APPROACHING BIRTH

Sally Inch is the author of *Birthrights* (reprinted by Green Print, London 1989). She has been a regular contributor to a number of journals, in particular the *Journal of the Royal Society of Medicine* and the *Journal of Maternal and Child Health*, and edited *Successful Breastfeeding — a handbook for midwives* for the Royal College of Midwives (London, 1988).

APPROACHING BIRTH

*Meeting the challenge
of labour*

Sally Inch

Illustrations by Joanne Acty

GREEN
PRINT

First published in 1989 by
Green Print
an imprint of The Merlin Press Ltd
10 Malden Road, London NW5 3HR

ISBN 1 85425 024 8

1 2 3 4 5 6 7 8 9 10: : 99 98 97 96 95 94 93 92 91 90 89

Printed in England by Biddles Ltd., Guildford
on recycled paper

For James

Acknowledgements

I could never have produced this book unaided — my thanks therefore go to:

My mother, Nora Cade, for reading through and commenting on the first draft and for typing additional material;

My children, James and Jenny, for their patience and their help with typing;

My husband, Steve, for his help with proof reading;

Kay Greenish, for commenting on the final text;

Joanne Acty for her care and attention in producing the drawings;

and all the women it has been my privilege to meet through NCT antenatal classes, many of whom have shared their experiences with subsequent classes in the form of labour reports, extracts of which have been used for this book (names, where used, have been changed to preserve anonymity further).

Contents

*Never does nature say one way
and wisdom another*

Satires, Juvenal, c.60 – c. 130 AD

Introduction

Too many women in Western societies still approach the birth of their child, an event which will colour and shape the remainder of their lives, inadequately prepared. Although this does not necessarily mean that the outcome cannot be satisfactory in psychological terms, many emerge from the experience much sadder as well as wiser. Yet there is no insurmountable reason why every woman should not be able to have the sort of birth she can look back on as the best she could achieve. For some this will not preclude regrets, but for all it could be a positive and enriching experience.

For the vast majority of women birth is a normal physiological process, and it could be for even more were they not exposed to unnecessary interventions.[1] This book is written with that fact in mind, and thus considers the ways in which a woman might try to ensure that her experience of labour remains within her perception of what she can cope with—a highly individual judgement!

However it also acknowledges that birth is never simply 'natural'. Any woman who gives birth does so within the context of the culture in which she has grown up. Her attitudes and expectations are culturally shaped and in all societies, from the most sophisticated to the most 'primitive', the birth process itself is surrounded and moulded by 'ritual and myth, injunctions, prohibitions and taboos'.[2]

The message that many modern British women receive from their society is that birth is mysterious, dangerous and painful.

This may in part have been influenced by the fact that more women in the past were physically less well equipped to cope with labour than their modern-day counterparts, as a result of inadequate nutrition in childhood (making bony deformities more common), poor nutrition in pregnancy, poor hygiene and other social privations. They have thus passed on the expectation that labour might not be straightforward.

It might also be due in part to the increasing medicalization of childbirth, as more and more (male) doctors have become involved in what was essentially and historically 'women's business'.[3]

The process of medicalization accelerated in the 1960s and 1970s as more and more Western women had their babies in hospital and were exposed to more and more interventions, many of which increased women's need for analgesics.[4] Many of these women then continued to live with the belief that analgesia was necessary 'in their case' because of the nature of labour, rather than because of the nature of the intervention. It has been said that 'Doctors succeed in tapping into a powerful combination of our oldest fears—"What if something goes wrong?" "What if I can't stand the pain?"—and our particularly modern beliefs that technology equals progress and the magic of obstetrical technology will guarantee a "better" or "perfect" baby.'[5]

The perspective is often reinforced by the fictional portrayal of childbirth in books and films, on radio and television, in which women are supine and distressed, with their tense and anxious attendants reacting as if this was appropriate behaviour. Very few women in Britain ever see a 'real' labour taking place in a calm and relaxed atmosphere before they come to experience labour for themselves.

This book is thus an attempt to dispel some of the myths that surround labour, particularly the view that women are powerless to affect their experience of it, that those who cope with labour without the need for drugs are 'just lucky', or that labour itself is such that most women will need drugs at some stage. However it is not a prescription for a painless labour, nor an exhortation to cope with labour without the use of pain-relieving techniques. Nor is it a criticism of women who have found drugs to be necessary, or of those who have elected to use them from the outset.

Moreover it is recognized that women use drugs in labour to help them cope with feelings other than pain. Deprived of a calm, private, supportive atmosphere in which she can focus her attention entirely on her labour, a woman may feel that only by removing the sensations of labour can she retain her dignity in the situation. In a labour ward atmosphere, in which a woman feels that she is 'having a baby in a stranger's drawing room',[6] she may choose to use drugs to enable her to maintain a sense of social control in her relationship with her attendants.

Nevertheless, women the world over do give birth without the aid of drugs; many because they have no alternative, but many because they do not expect to need them. This is particularly apparent if drug usage rates are compared in different Western industrial countries in which sophisticated pharmacological preparations are equally available. For example, at a time when the drug-usage rate in the UK was 95 per cent, it was 5 per cent in Holland.[7] This does not mean that Dutch women feel less in labour, but it does suggest that they have culturally induced expectations that their experiences in labour will come within the bounds of their minds' and bodies' ability to cope, and that these expectations are realized in practice.[8]

For most women labour is a challenge, but it is one that can be met with confidence in this age of information, where cultural expectations of birth are rooted more firmly in fact than in fiction.

Broadly speaking this book is divided into three sections; (1) what happens in labour; (2) what may be felt; and (3) how a woman can help herself to prepare and cope with the process of giving birth. This last aspect will include not only antenatal preparation for labour but 'setting the scene' in terms of the place of birth, birth attendants and the systems of care-giving that are available.

N.B.   I acknowledge that babies are either male or female, but as all mothers are female, I have, for the sake of clarity, referred to the baby as he, or him, throughout.

1 The Anatomy and Physiology of Labour

In order to begin to make sense of explanations of what they may feel in labour or do to help themselves, most women will need some understanding, not only of what happens, but where it happens within their bodies. Health care professionals often assume that pregnant women carry in their heads the same mechanistic model of the human body that they themselves have acquired through their years of study, and give their explanations accordingly. But women who do not share the health professionals' concept of anatomy and physiology are in much the same position as motorists who know nothing of the layout or inner workings of their car. Both are ill-equipped to enter into any discussion with an 'expert' who is suggesting anything from fine tuning to major modifications. Thus this chapter begins with the layout and functioning of the normal, pregnant, female body.

This drawing shows a non-pregnant adult woman, viewed from the side. Below the diaphragm, the stomach and intestines can be seen apparently filling the abdominal cavity. Beneath these structures is the small, non-pregnant uterus, just above the bladder.

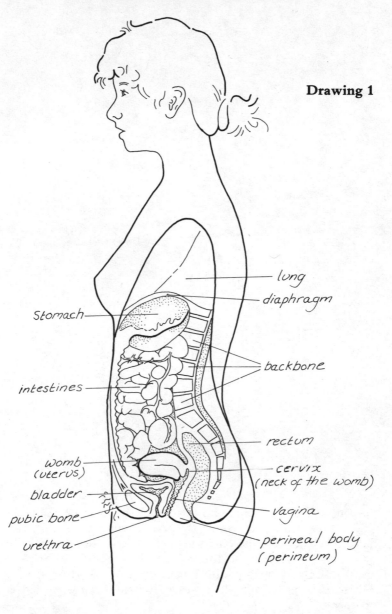

Drawing 1

lung

diaphragm

Stomach

backbone

intestines

rectum

womb
(uterus)

cervix
(neck of the womb)

bladder

pubic bone

vagina

urethra

perineal body
(perineum)

In contrast, this diagram shows an adult woman almost at the end of pregnancy. Everything shown in Drawing 1 is still there, but tucked around the enlarged uterus. It illustrates how the woman's body adapts to the growing baby, and also helps to explain some of the discomfort many women experience during pregnancy, including their need to empty their bladder frequently.

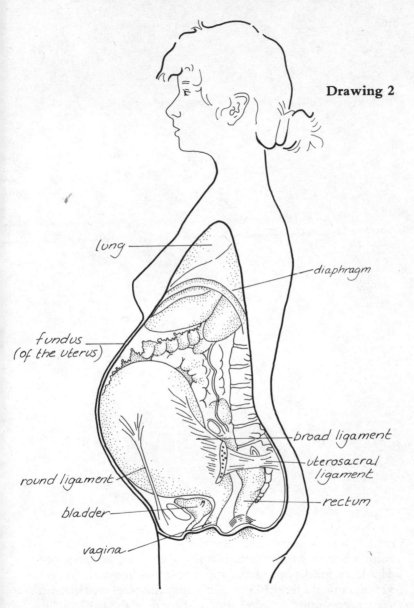

Drawing 2

lung

diaphragm

fundus
(of the uterus)

broad ligament

uterosacral
ligament

round ligament

bladder

rectum

vagina

Here we see a woman about half way through her pregnancy. The baby still has plenty of room to move about freely in the sac of amniotic fluid (the waters), and the placenta (afterbirth) still appears quite large relative to the size of the baby.

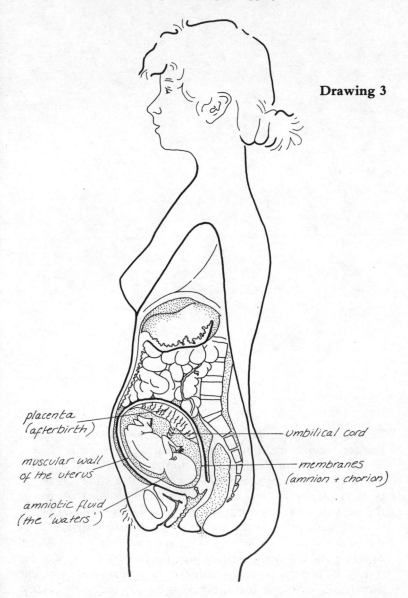

Drawing 3

placenta
(afterbirth)

muscular wall
of the uterus

amniotic fluid
(the 'waters')

umbilical cord

membranes
(amnion + chorion)

This diagram is similar to Drawing 2, but shows the uterus, bladder, vagina and bowel in section. The baby can be seen taking up most of the 'space' within the uterus, and is in the curled up, head down position which is most common at this point in pregnancy. If a line were drawn in, joining the top of the pubic bone to the junction of the spine and the top of the sacrum (the sacral promontory), it would be seen that most of the baby's head is above that line, and thus not yet 'engaged' in the pelvis. It can also be seen that the cervix (the neck of the uterus) is long and closed, with the plug of mucus (later 'the show') still within it. If this cervix were touched with a finger it would feel quite firm.

Drawing 4

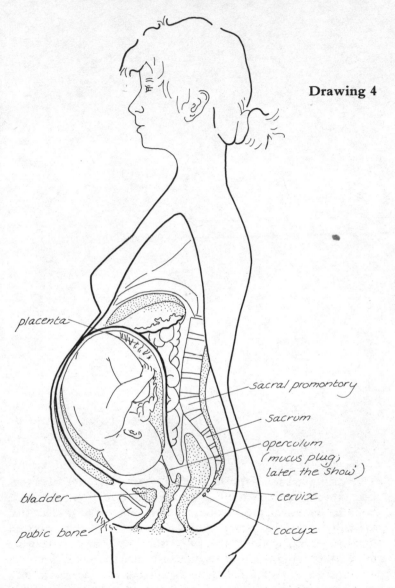

This diagram shows the mother and baby a couple of weeks later. In contrast to Drawing 4, a line drawn from the pubic bone to the sacral promontory would now make it clear that the baby's head has engaged in the pelvis. It can also be seen that the cervix, while still closed, is shorter. If this cervix were touched it would feel much softer than that shown in Drawing 4. (Engagement of the head is of interest to caregivers in a woman's first pregnancy, as it suggests that her pelvis is big enough for her baby to pass through easily).

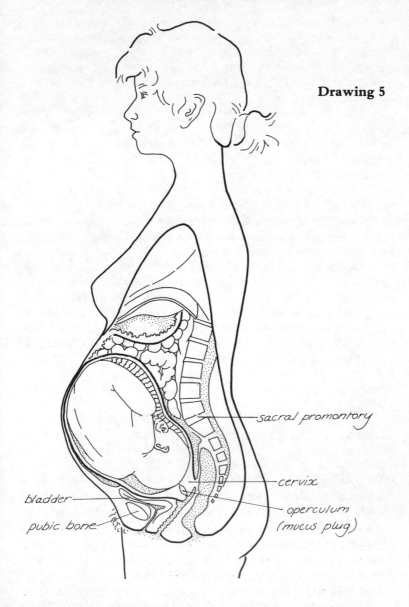

Drawing 5

sacral promontory

cervix

bladder

pubic bone

operculum
(mucus plug)

During the course of pregnancy the muscular uterus grows as the baby grows. It starts as an organ weighing about 2 oz and ends up weighing about 2 lbs. There are three layers of muscle in the wall of the uterus which, while not anatomically separate, have different functions. The longitudinal muscle fibres run from the cervix, up to the top (fundus) of the uterus and down the other side. (Some of them start half-way between the cervix and the fundus, run over the top and stop half-way down the other side.) When the longitudinal muscle fibres contract they shorten the uterus. They are therefore mainly used in the expulsive, second stage of labour.

The spiral or oblique muscle fibres also start at the cervix and run in all directions in the body of the uterus. When these contract during labour they play a major part in 'taking up' or shortening the elongated cervix had then dilating it until it is eventually wide enough to allow the baby's head to pass through and down the vagina without obstruction. At this point the cervix is said to be fully dilated. During and after the separation of the placenta the spiral fibres, by virtue of being entwined in a figure-of-eight fashion around the blood vessels supplying the placental site, help to reduce blood loss after the baby is born.

The circular fibres, as the name implies, pass in a horizontal manner around the uterus, mainly in the lower half of the uterus and the cervix. When these contract, they tend to close the cervix and inhibit activity of the lower part of the uterus in labour.

Although exercise in pregnancy has been shown to confer some benefit[1], it is not necessary (or possible) for the pregnant woman to take any particular form of exercise to ensure that the muscles of her uterus are physically prepared for labour. The uterine muscles 'take their own exercise' in the form of irregular, painless contraction and relaxation from the ninth or tenth week of pregnancy onwards (Braxton-Hicks contractions). These may be noticed by the pregnant woman and/or her care giver from about mid-pregnancy, and tend to become stronger and more noticeable as pregnancy progresses. (Many women, however, appear not to notice them at any time during their pregnancy.)

At the end of pregnancy/beginning of labour, the uterine

muscle exhibits a new ability; that of retraction. In all other muscles of the body, those involved in bending an arm, for example, contraction of the muscles is followed by complete relaxation of the muscles; the fibres of which are the same length and thickness both before and after the contraction. Retraction refers to the progressive shortening and 'fattening' of the muscle fibres as they contract and almost relax, rather like taking two steps forward and one backwards.

The net effect of this is to shorten the uterus from top to bottom, and this is first 'seen' as the cervix is gradually 'taken up', if this has not already happened in the last few weeks of pregnancy. Indeed, the division between the end of pregnancy and the onset of labour is often so blurred that it might be more helpful to think of labour as a continuation of a process, rather than a sudden event. The changes seen between Drawings 4 and 5, described as taking place in the last weeks of pregnancy, could equally well be used to illustrate the changes taking place at the beginning of labour.

When a woman is going into labour for the first time in her life, her cervix will usually become shortened before it starts to dilate. In subsequent labours the two processes may occur together.

Once the cervix has been 'taken up', continued contraction and retraction of the uterine muscles causes the cervix (or strictly speaking the cervical os) to start to dilate. If it could be viewed 'end on', the cervix would appear as a small circle, gradually getting bigger and bigger, until finally it was big enough to allow the baby's head to pass through (see Drawings 7 and 8).

The degree of dilatation of the cervix is assessed using a scale of 1 to 10 centimetres (see Drawing 6). This is done by the midwife during the course of an internal (vaginal) examination. She gently inserts (only) her first and middle fingers into the woman's vagina until she can feel the cervix. By parting her fingers within the 'circle' of the dilating cervix she gauges the number of centimetres between them.

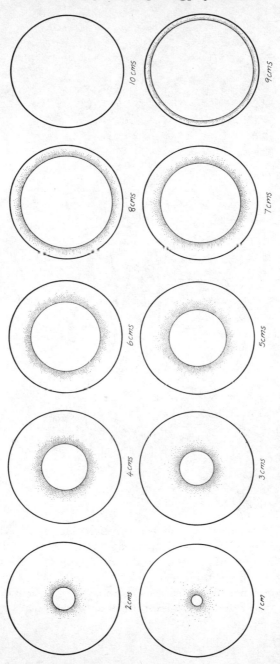

Drawing 6

Drawing 7

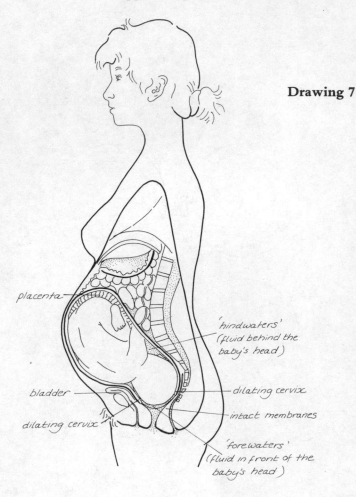

placenta

'hindwaters'
(fluid behind the
baby's head)

bladder

dilating cervix

dilating cervix

intact membranes

'forewaters'
(fluid in front of the
baby's head)

If the cervix were to dilate at a constant rate, say 1 centimetre per hour, it might be expected that full dilatation would be reached in 10 hours. Although this may sometimes be the case, in most instances the cervix dilates more slowly than this in early labour and the rate of dilatation increases as labour progresses. Most women therefore, will take longer to reach 5

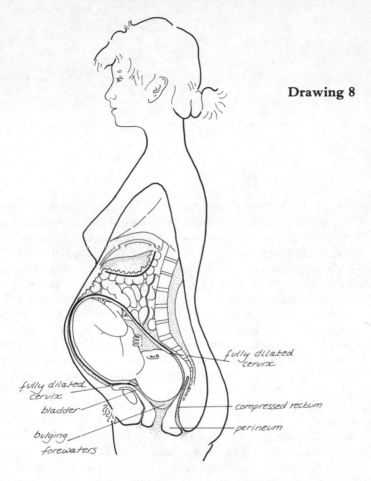

Drawing 8

fully dilated
cervix

fully dilated
cervix

bladder

bulging
forewaters

compressed rectum

perineum

centimetres dilatation than they will to reach full dilatation from 5 centimetres.

Once full dilatation has been reached, the first of the three stages of labour will have been completed. This takes, on average, 8–12 hours for a first labour, and 4–8 hours for subsequent labours.

As can also be seen from Drawings 7 and 8, the 'bag of waters' (the amniotic sac) surrounding the baby is still intact at the end of the first stage of labour. During labour the amniotic fluid surrounding the baby, which during pregnancy has acted as both a 'shock absorber' and a barrier to infection, takes on another equally important, hydrostatic function. As the uterus contracts, the pressure inside it also rises, and this rise in pressure extends to the baby's circulatory system within the placenta, umbilical cord, brain, skull and scalp. At the same time, the pressure of the amniotic fluid pressing on the outside of the baby also rises. Thus, while the bag of waters is intact, the rise in 'water' pressure outside compensates for the rise in pressure inside the baby. It also tends to reduce the downward pressure on the baby's skull bones, particularly when the head is engaged.[2]

During the second stage of labour, the muscles of the uterus are no longer 'pulling' open the cervix, but are 'pushing' the baby down and out of the vagina. At the same time the bladder is drawn up into the abdomen (to make more space and protect it from injury), the rectum is compressed and anything in it expelled, and the muscles that make up the wedge-shaped area between the rectum and vagina (the perineum) are slowly flattened out horizontally and vertically and pushed back, out of the way of the baby's head. Thinning out this area of muscle has the effect of lengthening the back wall of the vagina, and this helps to guide the baby's head round and forwards, following the curve of the sacrum (Drawing 9).

Drawing 9

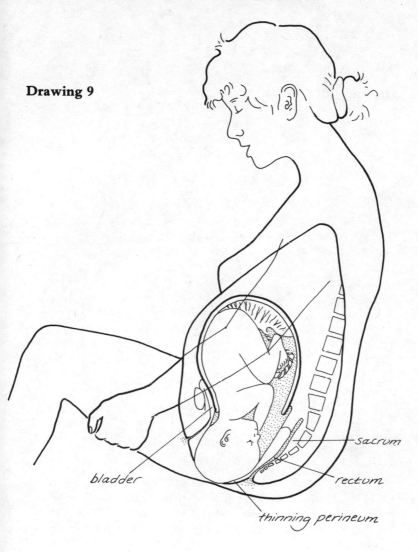

bladder

sacrum

rectum

thinning perineum

Drawing 10

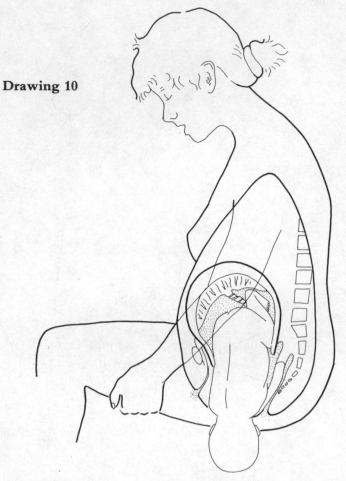

Once the baby is born, the second of the three stages of labour is complete. (See Drawings 10 and 11.) This takes, on average, 1–2 hours for a first labour, and 5–30 minutes for subsequent labours.

Drawing 11

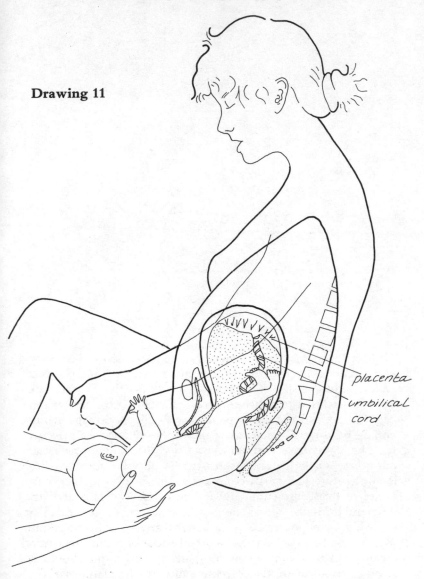

placenta

umbilical cord

The third, and final stage of labour is the separation and delivery of the placenta. As the baby is born, both the uterus and placenta rapidly reduce in size. (See Drawing 12). Once the placental site has been reduced to approximately half its original size, it can begin to peel off the inside of the uterus, like a postage stamp peeling off a rapidly deflating balloon. Sometimes the placenta separates completely with the contraction that delivers the baby, but more usually there is a short period of 'rest' after the baby is born before the uterus contracts again. The woman will be aware of this contraction, but it will probably feel somewhat different from the contractions of the second stage, and will probably be felt lower down in her abdomen. At this point the placenta will leave the upper part of the uterus and 'fall' into the lower part. If the woman is sitting on her haunches, or standing or kneeling, the placenta will very often fall out of the vagina by gravity. On other occasions the woman will need to bear down (as she did in the second stage) in order to expel it.

Drawing 12

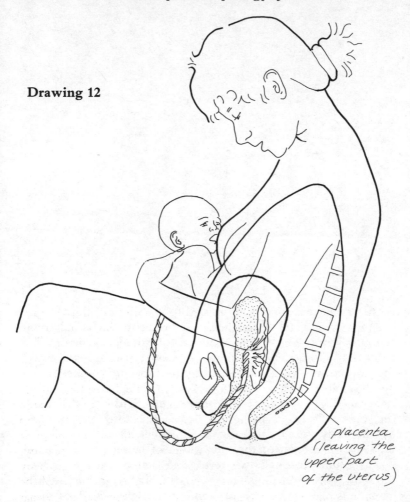

placenta
(leaving the
upper part
of the uterus)

At this point in a normal, unassisted (physiological) third stage, the baby would still be attached to the placenta via its pulsating umbilical cord. This would continue to provide oxygen to the baby until the placenta separated. It would also give the baby the opportunity to begin extra-uterine life with neither more nor less blood in his circulatory system than he needed. (See Drawing 13). Some time after the placenta had been delivered (in some cultures many hours elapse) the cord can be tied, usually fairly close to the baby, and then cut. (This physiologial sequence of events for the third stage of labour is still a rare sight in some hospitals, where routine 'active management' is thought to be preferable. Increasingly, however, women are extending their perception of labour beyond the birth of their babies, and many are now anxious to assume their share of the responsibility for the way in which the third stage of their labour is conducted.)

Recent observational research from Cambridge suggests that the third stage of labour takes on average 10–20 minutes in a first labour, and 5–10 minutes in subsequent labours.

Drawing 13

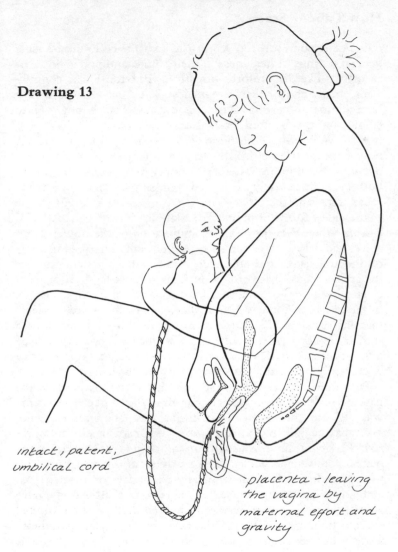

intact, patent,
umbilical cord

placenta – leaving
the vagina by
maternal effort and
gravity

How Labour Starts

It is not uncommon for women to experience low backache, general feelings of heaviness in their vagina and pelvic floor, or menstrual-like discomfort with strong Braxton-Hicks contractions, at the end of their pregnancy. They may also find they have a burst of 'nesting' activity a few days before they go into labour, but this is often a retrospective discovery!

In the very early labour period most women empty their lower bowel completely, either by having very loose, or small frequent bowel motions. The nerve supply to the uterus and lower bowel are quite closely connected, and stimulation of either may cause activity in the other. This fact is often made use of in one of the oldest forms of induction of labour; Castor Oil, Bath and Enema—the OBE. In this case stimulation of the bowel, from above and below, has been shown to produce a marked increase on the activity of the uterus at term,[3] and will often expedite the spontaneous onset of labour. This is most likely to be successful if a prior examination has revealed a soft, 'ripe' cervix. In the case of a labour which is starting spontaneously, it seems that increased uterine activity stimulates bowel activity in a similar fashion. As a result, most women do not need to be given enemas or suppositories in early labour, and this practice is gradually being abandoned in many hospitals.

For some women, the first sign that labour is close is the passage of 'the show'. This is the thick, jelly-like mucus that was sitting in the closed cervix during pregnancy (see Drawing 4). It may be light-brownish, purply-red or streaked with bright red. 'Having a show' is usually an indication that the cervix has begun to dilate and detach itself partly from the membranes. It may precede the onset of labour by a few days or a few hours, and sometimes it is passed after regular contractions have started. Occasionally it may be dislodged by a vigorous vaginal examination, in which case the fresh blood streaking may be slightly heavier. There should, however, be no real bleeding. (Bleeding in labour, as in pregnancy, requires medical attention.) A show is not always a reliable indication that labour is about to start, and unless the woman is anxious about it, it is not an event that needs to be reported to her care-givers.

... I awoke at 3.00 am with a contraction—nothing like as powerful as the Braxton-Hicks I'd been having for some time, but more like a period pain. Went to the loo and had a show. Contractions kept coming every five minutes—not very strong and I went back to bed to read a book. A little later I decided I'd better clear the decks in case this was the real thing ... Activity seemed to bring on contractions, which got stronger but no closer together, and at 5.00 am I woke Peter ... At 6.45 am, when the midwife called I was 5 centimetres dilated ...

Prior to the onset of labour the baby's chin is in most cases tucked into his chest, so that the top/back of his head fits snugly into the cervix (see Drawing 5). When this happens, the fluid in front of the baby's head (the forewaters) is largely cut off from the remainder of the fluid (the hindwaters). This event reduces the pressure applied to the forewaters each time the uterus contracts, and helps to keep them intact despite strong contractions. Thus the closed system of amniotic fluid can continue to perform its physiological function in labour—that of equalizing the pressure applied to all parts of the baby, his cord and placenta—in most cases until the end of the first stage.[4,5]

In one study of 517 women, 62 of them (12 per cent) still had the membranes intact at delivery.[4] (Being born in a 'caul', i.e. in the intact sac of membranes, was once considered to protect the individual from death by drowning!) However, in some cases the membranes will rupture spontaneously quite early in labour, and even before the contractions start. This is more common when the baby is lying head down but with his back towards his mother's back rather than towards her front (a posterior position). If the 'break' in the bag of waters is behind the baby's head (a hindwater leak) it will probably trickle out fairly slowly, and many women in this situation, particularly if they have been subject to slight incontinence at the end of pregnancy, are unsure whether they are leaking urine or amniotic fluid (liquor), since amniotic fluid has very little colour and very little smell at the end of pregnancy. The easiest way for a woman to tell the difference is for her to empty her bladder completely, put on a sanitary pad and see whether or not she continues to get wet. If she decides that she is leaking liquor, or she is still unsure, she should contact her midwife or hospital. If the waters break in front of the baby's head, (a forewater leak) a woman is likely to be in much less doubt as to what has happened, as she will probably be aware of a small 'gush' (of about a teacupful) rather than a 'leak'. This is more likely to occur after the contractions have started, but may happen quite early on in labour. If it happens as the first event, contractions usually start fairly quickly afterwards, unlike those in the case of a hindwater leak.

When spontaneous rupture of the membranes occurs early in labour, it is more likely to happen late at night or early in the morning, i.e. when the woman is still in bed (not at the supermarket checkout!). For this reason it is advisable to protect the mattress in some way from about the thirty-sixth week of pregnancy onwards. The baby will be surrounded by about two pints of fluid at the end of pregnancy (term), and although it is highly unlikely that all this will be lost at once, even a small cupful can make a mattress quite wet. The chief reason for reporting the actual or suspected rupture of the membranes to the hospital/midwife, particularly if contractions have not started, is that the longer the interval between the membrane rupture and delivery, the greater the risk of infection of the amniotic fluid. Opinions vary as to how long it is safe to wait for contractions to start before inducing labour, but most doctors will want to give antibiotics as a precaution if the membranes have been ruptured longer than 12–24 hours.

For most women, labour will 'begin' with contractions. As noted earlier, the onset of labour is the culmination of a process that has been going on for some time; it is rarely perceived as an 'event', like turning on a light switch. Thus very few women know the precise time that their labour started, all they can tell their care-givers is the time at which they were first aware of contractions coming at regular intervals. This will depend to a large extent on what the woman is doing. If she is asleep, or deeply engrossed in some activity, she is less likely to notice early contractions than a woman who is awake but doing very little. It is not uncommon, however, for a woman to have one or more episodes of regular contractions towards the end of pregnancy which are fairly weak and do not become progressively longer and stronger, and then cease altogether, having lasted possibly several hours.

'True' labour contractions may therefore be recognized by the fact that not only do they occur at regular intervals, but that as time goes by the intervals reduce and the contractions feel stronger (and are in fact dilating the cervix). Thus when deciding when to call the midwife, a woman should take into consideration not only the frequency of her contractions, but also their length and strength. Long, strong, contractions occurring at seven-minute intervals may well be taking the woman more quickly towards the birth of her baby than short, weak contractions every five minutes.

Some women will first notice their contractions when they are coming only at intervals of 20–30 minutes, and lasting 30 seconds or so; others will be unaware until they have (gradually) increased to intervals of 5–10 minutes, lasting 45–50 seconds.

We had a very convincing false alarm nine days earlier, with regular contractions from 2.00 am to 7.00 am; so when contractions started on Friday morning, also at 2.00 am, I was thrilled, but cautiously so. I stayed in bed, half dozing, with very regular but not very strong contractions every 10 minutes, until Jim woke up and we decided to have some breakfast. By 6.00 am contractions lasting 45–50 seconds every five minutes prompted me to ring the midwife. I found that if I knelt upright against two beanbags I could relax completely with my head supported during contractions. By 6.50 am I was having extremely strong contractions every few minutes, and as I began to doubt my ability to go on coping, I suddenly felt the first urge to push . . .

Established Labour

. . . There was a nice gradual build-up of contractions and I went through the first part of labour saying 'another one!' with pleasure . . .

Towards the end of the first stage the contractions may be 2–3 minutes apart, lasting between 50 and 60 seconds, and as second stage approaches they may in some cases occur every 1½–2 minutes and last for 60–90 seconds, feeling to the woman as if they are almost continuous. In some labours contractions may vary in strength from one contraction to the next, and some women may experience contractions that reach a peak, start to fade and then recur without a 'break' (twin-peaked contractions).

> . . . At 11.30 am I decided to get up on the bed and start concentrating. After that they accelerated. The more upright I was, the easier they were to cope with. I absolutely flopped between contractions—no need to work at relaxation! The head was descending slowly—sometimes I could feel it going down, which was lovely . . .

Sometimes the contractions may die down for a short period before the second stage starts, and when they resume they are different in quality as the expulsive urge builds up. Sometimes the first and second stages seem to overlap, and the urge to push may begin before the cervix is fully dilated. (This seems to be less likely if the woman has been more or less upright during the first stage.)

As the first stage unfolds and the cervix dilates steadily, the whole process seems to become progressively more efficient as contractions become longer, stronger and closer together. During this period, as the second stage approaches, many women experience sensations that have not been a feature of the early part of their labour.

As the uterus contracts more strongly, it also begins to rise up during contractions. As can be seen from Drawing 7, the stomach is immediately above the contracting uterus, and will itself be pushed upwards. If there is much food in the stomach it is not uncommon for the woman to vomit at this stage. Once the stomach contents have been expelled, it is unlikely that nausea will persist.

> . . . Contractions began to need a higher level of breathing and that was when I started worrying how long things would go on, but I felt sick and hoped this meant transition . . .

As the baby's head stimulates the cervix and the nerve-endings in the pelvic floor, it is sometimes the case that the muscles of the upper, inner thigh are also stimulated and the woman's legs may begin to shake. (Sometimes her whole body shakes). Shaking is less likely if the woman is using her legs for support or to walk about. If she is at rest, gentle massage of the thighs may help; but the shaking is not usually distressing, just surprising. The least helpful approach is to try and keep them from shaking by tightening the muscles, as many other muscles will become tense in the process.

Women who have not experienced backache during the first part of their labour may find it develops as the second stage approaches. Both this, and the gradual build up of rectal pressure are due to the backwards pressure of the baby's head as it follows the curve of the mother's sacrum, back, round and forwards. (See Drawings 8 and 9). Sometimes the sensation of rectal pressure occurs quite suddenly and the woman may feel as if she wants to empty her bowels. This may, in fact, be the case, but is more likely to be due to compression of the empty rectum between the baby's head and the sacrum as the head descends.

> . . . I think in retrospect that all this happened much more quickly than either the midwife or I expected. I must have gone from 7 cm to full dilatation in about an hour, because the next thing that happened was that I emptied my bowels—and the midwife suddenly asked if I wanted to push. I said no, but was examined to find that I was fully dilated . . .

Some women find that they move to a different level of consciousness in advanced labour, as if they were entering a world of their own, in which time ceases to have meaning. They may appear to their companions to be in a trance-like state, or even asleep between contractions. In this state women seem to escape from the restraints of social conventions, and respond entirely to something deep within them. They move and act according to their 'instincts', finding positions that suit them, and which are also likely to be the most efficient physiologically.[6] It seems that a woman's entry to this state is connected with a particular hormonal balance, the exact nature of which is not yet known, but in which endorphins (neurohormones with a morphine-like function) play a major role. These 'endogenous opiates' seem to suppress pain and anxiety and induce a sense of well-being, so that the woman can not only work with her labouring body to its best advantage but her perception of labour (powerful though it is) stays within the limits of what she feels she can cope with. When this state of 'hormonal balance' is reached, mind and body seem to function as one harmonious unit.

> . . . So we sat or lay in this quiet little pink cave, (it really felt like the inside of an egyptian tomb—sacrosanct and still) nobody talking at all, lights dim, no fuss. Oddly I could even—in well-coped-with contractions—lift my mind away from my body in a kind of self-hypnosis, and got not sleepy or dopy but somehow onto a very low tick-over rate (a kind of natural and unconfused version of pethidine) . . .

However, a variety of circumstances can affect a woman's ability to reach this state, and unfortunately many women labour without the full help of their natural 'opiates'. In this situation they are more likely to experience feelings of disorientation, (possibly because they are half in and half out of 'real time'), irritability, panic or desperation; all of which are consequences of the increased stress of coping with the increasingly powerful sensations of labour without being able to 'tune in' effectively to their inner resources. (This period of labour is dealt with in greater detail in Chapter 2.)

> . . . Getting dressed to go to the hospital was frightful; every time I tried to do up a button or pull up my tights I had an almighty contraction or felt as if I had to rush to the loo—thinking I was in for another long hard slog it didn't occur to me that I might be wanting to push already . . . I also had this odd feeling of being shut away from every one else, reinforced by the fact that an irrational bit of me felt much 'further' on than it seemed I was; correctly as it turned out!

The Approaching Birth

Technically the second stage begins at the point at which the cervix is completely, or fully, dilated, but this precise moment in time may go unnoticed unless a vaginal examination is done. There are a number of external signs that indicate to the attending midwife that the woman is entering the second stage. As with the concept of the 'beginning of labour' it is probably more helpful to regard the second stage as the culmination of the process rather than an event having a definable beginning.

For the woman, the transition from the first to the second stage is often accompanied by new sensations. A build up of rectal pressure (as discussed earlier) is often a feature, and she may find that she is 'catching' her breath or grunting with contractions. (The waters may break spontaneously around this time; they are no longer 'needed' in quite the same way as in the first stage). Often the contractions feel qualitatively different in the second stage, as they change from drawing up the cervix to pushing the baby down and out of the uterus and vagina. Often they space out a little, perhaps occuring at 3-minute intervals where before they were coming every 1½–2 minutes. By the time the baby's head has reached the woman's pelvic floor, where it distends her vagina and triggers the release of more oxytocin* (the Ferguson reflex[7]). The woman will probably find that she experiences a strong expulsive urge at the height (not the beginning) of contractions and find herself using her abdominal muscles to help her uterine muscles to deliver her baby.

> . . . At last there was enough of a break to change position and I flopped right over the bean bag so that my back was horizontal. I had time for two gulps of water, through a straw, before I started to push the baby out. The midwife said she could see the membranes over the head, and a few moments later they went on their own and then I felt the head crowning—painful, but marvellous because I knew we were nearly there . . . the head was born followed by the

---

*Oxytocin is a hormone, chiefly concerned in labour with stimulation of contractions of the uterus.

longest wait for ages, for the next contraction to push the body out. Absolute bliss and utter physical relief as the little body slithered forward onto my quickly seated lap . . .

In some women the expulsive urge is mild or absent, in which case contractions are often felt to be more like first-stage contractions. Although the second stage may be longer if the woman does not exert any voluntary effort to help her uterus push out her baby, he will be born just as surely, as the uterus does most of the expulsive work in all labours.

. . . I think stage two lasted about an hour and a half, shorter by about half an hour than my first labour. As with that one I felt no urge to push that the books universally speak of, only this time I knew I had to, and I knew how to. Contractions were every 5 minutes, sharp but short—however a few good ones came along and with the midwife's excellent coaching I was able to push to good effect . . . unfortunately clearing my bowels at the same time, but no one minded, so I didn't!

Normal vaginal deliveries are possible even in women with spinal cord injuries that have resulted in paralysis.[8] In contrast some women find the second stage totally overwhelming, but for the majority it is experienced as a powerful surge of energy.

. . . It's true that second stage contractions, when you're pushing, don't exactly hurt, but they do shock by the immense force of an entirely new sensation . . .

The second stage is often characterized by a sudden need to grasp something or someone, and in many cultures labouring women have a rope suspended from the ceiling or rafters to hang onto, a stake driven into the ground to hold onto, or post or wall against which to lean. In almost all of the cultures studied by Naroll[9] the woman was assisted by several female helpers, who provided direct physical support. Women who have been standing or walking in labour often feel the need to bend their knees as they hold on. (Standing, squatting and kneeling were the commonest positions adopted by women in the seventy-six cultures studied by Naroll,[9] with a sitting position being almost as common. Sixty-two out of the seventy-six thus used 'upright' positions).

> . . . By now Michael was holding me tightly, so I pushed her out held in his arms. Absolutely overwhelming experience—quite orgasmic. Pushing wasn't painful at all because the pushing blotted out anything else. It was marvellous; I really felt her head come out—I never believed I could stretch so well . . .

In many women the second stage progresses slowly and steadily, so that gradually more and more of the baby's head can be seen until finally the whole head emerges. During this time the muscles of the perineum have time to thin out and stretch and the woman may experience a hot, burning sensation round the entrance to the vagina, which reaches its peak as the widest part of the baby's head is born (crowning). Often there is then a pause (1–2 minutes) while the final second stage contraction is awaited—the one that will deliver the baby's body. Some women however, having experienced a straightforward first stage, often in a tranquil and supportive atmosphere[10], are suddenly overtaken by a sense of panic. This is often accompanied by feelings of thirst, a sudden burst of muscular energy and powerful uterine contractions, possibly originating in the cervical region, and rapidly spreading downwards in a wave-like fashion. In a very short space of time (sometimes only one or two contractions) the baby is born.[11] Despite the lack of 'time' for the perineum to stretch, perineal damage is very rare. This powerful 'fetus ejection reflex', although rarely seen in 'environmentally disturbed labours', can sometimes be triggered by sudden cooling or by fear, such as the threat of a forceps delivery.[10, 11]

> . . . I managed to stop pushing, when told, quite easily, probably because I disliked the pushing feeling so much and was only too ready to stop. The head was born—an absolutely amazing sight, with silver fair hair, especially after all the pictures I'd seen in which the baby's head was always covered in black hair! Almost immediately came the mightiest contraction of them all, terrifyingly strong and

the baby catapulted along the bed. I knew at once that he was all right—I could see he was so pink and whole . . .

After Birth

If the mother reaches down to take hold of her baby as he is born, he will follow the continuation of the curve of her sacrum onto her abdomen or into her arms. Otherwise, the baby will rest on the floor/ground, having either slid there because the mother's buttocks are touching or very close to the ground, or having been lowered there by an attendant as he emerged. A mother who gave birth on all fours or kneeling might then sit back on her heels to look at and touch her baby, and one who stood or squatted might then sit down. Unless the birth attendant intervenes, (by giving the baby to the mother), the mother will be upright before she takes her baby in her arms, either because she was already upright or because she has had to bring herself into an upright position. Thus even a woman who has given birth lying on her back or on her side will be upright after the birth, and this will ensure that gravity can assist in the delivery of the placenta. The uninterrupted flow of blood through the intact umbilical cord will ensure that the baby continues to receive oxygenated blood (should he need it) until the placenta separates[12] and will allow any necessary volume adjustments to be made to the baby's circulatory system.[13] It will also reduce the likelihood of the baby's blood cells (from the blood in the placenta) entering the mother's circulation in sufficient quantity to stimulate her body to make antibodies, if she is Rhesus negative and her baby Rhesus positive.[14] Even more importantly, it will allow placental separation to take place without interruption, reducing the risk of bleeding and of the placenta being retained.[15, 16]

The sight and sound of the baby, as well as skin to skin contact, seem to facilitate the delivery of the placenta by stimulating the uterus to contract strongly.[17, 18] Gravity, coupled in some cases with the mother's bearing down efforts, is usually all that is then necessary for placental delivery.

Putting the baby to the breast will also cause the release of the hormone that makes the uterus contract (oxytocin), but there is no reason to suppose that this is a necessary or integral part of the process of placental separation. Few babies are actually ready to feed, as opposed to having a slippery nuzzle, immediately after the birth. The majority will be ready within the first hour and almost all within two hours of birth,[19] but the cue should ideally come from the baby.

2 Pain in Labour

Pain in labour is neither necessary nor inevitable. However, at a time when standard practice dictated that most women should receive large amounts of narcotic drugs during the first stage of labour, and general anaesthetics at the end of the second stage as a matter of course, pain in labour was *assumed* to be inevitable. From the 1930s onwards this assumption began to be questioned, and from some quarters came the assertion that antenatal training in methods based on Pavlov's concepts of conditioned reflexes would permit women to experience 'painless childbirth'. As it became apparent that psychoprophylaxis and self-hypnosis were not the universal panacea, many professionals were confirmed in their belief that it was appropriate to warn women that labour would be painful; not to do so was felt to be 'dishonest'.

In fact it is just as unhelpful to tell a woman that labour will be painful as to tell her that it will not. If she has been told 'labour is not painful' she may be unable to cope if she does experience pain. On the other hand if she has been told 'labour is painful' she is likely to be in a state of tension, waiting for the pain. This diffuse state will tend to increase the intensity of the (new) sensations of labour and may bring her defence ('fight-or-flight') mechanisms into operation. (See page 47 for more detail.) The consequent release of adrenalin may be sufficient to stimulate the circular fibres of the uterus to contract and try to close the cervix, while the longitudinal and oblique muscle fibres are trying to open it. This tug-of-war rapidly produces a state

of abnormal tension in the walls of the uterus, which is registered by the receptors specific for that form of stimulation, and
correctly interpreted as pain. In this situation the woman has
involuntarily fulfilled the prophecy, and the vicious circle of
fear-tension-pain (as described by Dick-Read[1]) has been set up.

Many factors may trigger this unhappy state of affairs, both
in pregnancy and labour. Health professionals and others persist
in referring to 'pains' when they mean contractions. Some antenatal classes teach relaxation but stress the availability of drugs
'for when it gets too bad' or 'when the breathing isn't enough'.
In many hospitals the suggestion of pain is conveyed by the
atmosphere of labour and delivery rooms, which look like oper-
ating theatres, and by the attitudes of doctors, midwives, friends
and relatives. If they all believe in pain, then they are likely to
suggest, expect or even presume pain. Upon the highly recep-
tive mind of a woman in labour, sympathy (as opposed to
empathy), exhortations to 'be brave' or even 'not to be a
martyr', are all powerful pain producers.

The sensations of labour are hard to describe, but 'painful' is
often far from appropriate as a description. A crude measure of
the prevalence of pain, in societies where women have the
option of using pharmacological methods of pain relief, might
be the extent to which they are used; but in fact this might
reveal less about what they felt than about how they coped (or
were enabled to cope) with what they felt. When different
societies throughout the world are compared, it becomes apparent that the extent to which women expect, experience or
express pain in labour varies considerably. In some there is a
cultural recognition that pain is not inevitable, even to the extent
of having two distinct words for labour, one to describe 'pain
in labour' and one for 'labour' alone.[2, 3]

... I had to have some stitches which seemed to take forever, and
when he pulled a hair it seemed more painful than anything else I'd
felt all day. Pain is certainly a strange thing, it has so many different
forms. Certainly the pain of labour is very hard to grasp because it is
there and yet it disperses so quickly between each contraction. It is
the panic and loss of control that is most distressing ...

Since the sensations of labour are inevitably subjective, perhaps the only way to ascertain what women feel is to ask as many as possible. In a survey of 128 women who had attended antenatal classes (and who were therefore a highly selected group), 31 per cent said that they felt no pain at all in labour, and a further 49 per cent said that such pain as they experienced was tolerable and did not require any analgesia. Twelve per cent said they had been given drugs before they had felt the need for them and only 8 per cent had asked for pain relief.[4]

Except for a very small, perhaps unfortunate (see p. 45), minority of women who feel practically nothing when in labour, women who are not feeling pain are certainly feeling something. Many describe the sensations of labour as 'incredibly powerful', 'strong' or 'intense'; 'a tremendous surge of physical energy'. Others register the power of the contractions as heat; 'like sitting beside a hot oven, with the door slowly opening and then closing again'; or 'It felt as if I had a warm fire inside me; I could feel the glow as each contraction came'. Still others experience contractions 'like a tight band around the pelvis'. Some women find language so inadequate as a means of describing what they feel that they instead use colour and shape to convey the experience.

For the majority of women the contraction is felt mostly just above the pubic bone, which is where the cervix is. Others are aware predominantly of backache, or a feeling of heaviness in the thighs. Although the contractions are initiated at the top of the uterus (the fundus) they radiate downwards to the point at which they have their effect; the cervix. It is not uncommon for women to express surprise when they first feel contractions, having expected to feel them 'much higher up'.

The words used to determine what a woman feels are important. If a woman who considers that she has never experienced any real pain in her life (e.g. toothache, arthritis, broken limbs) is asked how painful her childbirth was by comparison with other painful experiences she has had, she is likely to report, if she had any pain, that childbirth was the most painful experience she had ever had. This was in fact what most of the 75 women questioned by researchers Davenport-Slack and Boylan[5] reported. Yet when these same women were asked to describe childbirth in terms of a range of 'extremely painful' to 'not painful at all', only 27 per cent put labour in the former category. In another survey of 141 women, who were asked to rate their childbirth experience on a scale from 'no pain' (through 'mild/discomforting/distressing/horrible') to 'excrutiating', twenty-three per cent of those having a first baby (primigravidae) and eleven per cent of those having a second or subsequent baby (multigravidae) had scores in the top third of the range; and twenty-four per cent of multigravidae and nine per cent of primigravidae had scores in the bottom third of the range.[6] (The women in both these studies were a representative sample of the hospital population; some had been to antenatal classes and some had not.)

Thus it would appear that the degree to which women experience pain varies very widely, and on a scale from one to ten, some will be at the top, some at the bottom and most somewhere in the middle. Thus to tell women, without qualification, that 'labour is painful' is not only unhelpful, but untrue.

Investigators have also found that a woman's reaction to her experience of labour varies enormously, and women's reports of positive and rewarding childbirth experiences are often not correlated with the presence or absence of pain.

> ... In retrospect the experience of childbirth gives a sense of achievement I imagine difficult to find in anything else. I may say at the time I didn't enjoy it and wondered whether towards the end of the first stage I was being a masochist doing without drugs ...

A woman who reports no pain at all in labour may not find the experience satisfactory. If she has been unaware of her labour until the moment of birth is almost upon her, she may be in a state of some shock following the baby's birth because she was totally unprepared for the event. Even those who have been aware of their labour in time to adjust psychologically, may complain that 'it was all too quick'. Conversely, women who do report having felt some pain, but who also feel the experience to have been satisfying, often try to qualify the admission of pain. They may use terms such as 'functional pain'[7], 'pain with a purpose' or 'round pain'; or they may say 'yes, there was pain, but it didn't matter'. These women seem to have made a distinction (albeit unconsciously) between the pain of injury (referred to by some as organic pain[7]) and functional pain which inflicts no injury and is accompanied by 'a sense of ease, even satisfaction . . . when it has passed'.[7] The parallel may be drawn between the pain that is felt when other physiological needs are not met, and is a warning signal that these needs, such as emptying the bladder or bowel, must be satisfied. Functional pain in labour, it may be similarly argued, is a signal that the muscles of the cervix and vagina are somehow resisting the process of labour.[7] Women who are able to heed this functional warning signal and respond to it by decreasing their muscular resistance to the process, are likely to report subsequently that they did feel some pain, but that they were able to cope with it. Forty-nine per cent of those in the study by Hommel mentioned earlier felt this way (80 per cent in this study coped with labour without needing analgesia.)[4] The fact that for many women the presence or absence of pain has little to do with whether or not they view their childbirth as a positive experience, highlights the importance of their ability to *cope* with what they experience, rather than focusing exclusively on *what* they experience. It may be that a lack of understanding of this point is what prompts some professionals to reach for analgesics as a 'first resort' rather than a 'last resort', on the assumption that what a woman wants, primarily, is to feel no pain. This may indeed be true for some women, but the fact that so many women who have epidural anaesthesia (and thus no pain at all) nevertheless regard their labour experience as unsatisfactory[19, 20] suggests that satisfaction has little to do with the absence of pain.

Anyone who has ever watched or played a fast and furious game of rugby/football/hockey etc. will know the difference between pain as a side effect of a strenuous activity willingly undertaken and the pain of suffering. If the joy of playing far outweighs the incidental bruises, the player will not be grateful for a 'treatment' that removes the ability to enjoy the game. This analogy assumes that the player understands the rules and knows what is involved in playing. The same degree of injury might be perceived quite differently by an unprepared and/or unwilling participant.

... It is quite impossible to put into words the emotions experienced in those next few moments, so I won't try. One doesn't forget the pain of labour as some people suggest, I can still recall it vividly now, but the moment of birth is so magical that I would go through that labour many times over to experience the moment of childbirth again, and that is something one can only know after the event ...

However even willing players would probably prefer to do without the bruises if they could do so and still enjoy the game, and a number of factors have been shown to influence both whether a woman experiences any pain, and her ability to cope with her labour if she does.

Factors that Influence Pain Perception

Perhaps the most potent pain producer is fear. Situations creating fear or anxiety awaken the primitive defence reaction and cause adrenalin and noradrenalin to be released into the bloodstream. These hormones result in diffuse changes in the body, in particular to the blood supply to individual organs and the state of activity of the muscles. The blood supply is reduced to those organs not required for defence (stomach, gut, uterus etc.) and diverted to those that are; heart, lungs and skeletal muscles, preparing the individual for running away or standing ground and fighting.

The fact that the uterus is actively contracting in labour does not alter the changes that take place in response to fear; and the blood supply to the uterus is decreased in spite of the work it is doing. The fact that pain can be produced by asking a muscle to work with too little oxygen is well known (e.g. angina, intermittent claudication) and can be simply demonstrated by rapidly opening and closing the fingers of one hand whilst restricting the blood supply at the wrist with the other.

The other effect of fear on the uterus, namely stimulation of the circular fibres of the uterus, has been discussed earlier (see p. 42). This mechanism, by which fear or anxiety damps down the muscular activity of the body of the uterus whilst causing the circular fibres to try and close the cervix,[8] is of benefit to some mammals, who can, if delivery is not imminent, cause labour to slow down or stop so that they can move to safer, quieter surroundings.[9] In other mammals, activation of this mechanism considerably increases the number of deliveries that require veterinary assistance, often with a corresponding rise in the perinatal mortality rate.[10] In labouring women, activation of this mechanism can produce a range of effects, from the dampening down of contractions as they move from one environment to another (usually home to hospital) through to inco-ordinate uterine action in which strong contractions produce much pain and little progress.

Most women face the prospect of labour, particularly their first, with some anxiety, and indeed this may be of value to them particularly if it leads to behaviour that will ultimately prepare them for the experience.[11] However, high anxiety levels exhibited in pregnancy, may result in a self-fulfilling prophecy in labour, if the woman is not enabled to confront her fears and receive the help she needs to face labour with confidence.[12, 13]

Simple, unopposed muscle contraction does not in itself produce pain. The only pain receptors in the abdomen are those that detect excessive tension in, or tearing of, the tissues. The intestine and uterus can be handled or moved without any sensation of pain, but stretching (or tearing) of these structures can result in considerable pain and shock. The pain perceived in labour must therefore result from one or both of these specific stimuli. Thus the functional pain referred to earlier can be seen to result from excessive stretching in the case of an over-full bladder, the increased pressure on muscles that do not 'give' sufficiently during a contraction, or pressure exerted on the contracting uterus itself. In this latter case the pressure may come from a full bladder below (hence the need to empty the bladder at intervals during labour) or tense abdominal muscles above. This type of pain can be simulated by strongly contracting the biceps muscle of the upper arm and then pressing hard upon it with the fingers of the other hand. To a lesser degree holding the breath in the first stage of labour, or trying to take deep breaths against a strongly contracting uterus, may produce this sort of pain.

A woman who is able to approach labour without fear (as opposed to slight apprehension), to relax her voluntary muscles in response to contractions and to breathe appropriately in labour is less likely to create a state of excessive tension in the muscles of her uterus. (These three elements are addressed in any good antenatal course).

No woman can alter the shape of her pelvis or the size of her baby by the way she behaves in labour, but she may be able to affect the way in which her uterus contracts, and how she perceives the contraction. The way in which 'fear-tension-pain' cycle affects the uterus has already been discussed, but uterine action can also be affected by the position(s) that the woman adopts in labour. It ought to be axiomatic that a woman in labour should be free to move around and adopt whatever position affords her the greatest comfort. Unfortunately a great many women are constrained from doing this; by machinery (drips, monitors etc), by furniture and space in the labour room, by professionals who feel that a woman in labour 'belongs' in bed or by conventions that make it difficult for the woman to do other than that which she feels she 'ought' to do, or is expected of her.

Many women labouring in a supportive, permissive environment, instinctively adopt positions which facilitate their labour. They adopt them because they find them comfortable, not because they are thinking clearly about the mechanics of labour, but generally speaking what is comfortable is also mechanically advantageous. (For example, a woman who is experiencing backache in labour because her baby is positioned with his back towards her back (a posterior position), may find comfort in an all fours (hands and knees) position. Coincidentally this is also the position that is most likely to encourage the baby to rotate to an anterior position).

> . . . even the tedious business of repairing my tear didn't detract from the satisfaction (not quite the right word) we felt at the way labour had gone. My overall feelings are of being totally relaxed (mentally as much as physically) and in control. The ability to change the tempo of the contractions by using different postures, and the very positive feeling of pushing the baby out without any wasted effort made me feel in charge of events . . .

Part of a large Latin-American collaborative study[14] involved allowing women to choose their own position in labour and documenting what they did. Ninety-five per cent of the women studied chose to stand, sit, or walk. When these women were compared, as a group, with another group who 'volunteered' to lie down, the active group reported much less pain.

Another part of the study looked at what happened to the uterus when the woman adopted different positions. It was found[15] that the effectiveness of the contractions was much greater; the efficiency and rate of cervical dilatation was improved although the frequency of the contractions remained the same, when the women were not lying supine. It has since been suggested[7] that in reclining positions, the uterus must contract against gravity to elongate and move itself forward, and that this wastes much-needed energy. Other researchers have demonstrated that upright positions are associated with a reduced need for analgesics.[16, 17]

It may be that what is important is not that a woman should adopt any particular position, but that she should be free to choose the position in which she is most comfortable. (It should be borne in mind that for five per cent of the women in the Latin-American study the most comfortable position was lying down). But being free to choose implies a range of options from which to choose. This range might be increased if women received specific instruction and tried out different positions antenatally, and if their attendants were similarly instructed.[18] Saying 'do whatever you like' to a woman in labour is often not as helpful to her as saying 'would you like to try . . .' or 'have you considered . . .' followed by a specific suggestion (always with the proviso that the woman can decline if it doesn't appeal to her).

Another factor, discussed in Chapter 1, which appears to be related to the perception of pain, is the degree to which a woman is able to manufacture and release endorphins, the body's natural 'opiates'. The situations in which the kind of behaviour described on pages 35–6 is most likely to occur are also the situations in which research has suggested women are less likely to use analgesic drugs. This may be because the way in which a stimulus is interpreted is as important as the stimulus itself.

This in turn is likely to be affected by the mental state of the woman.

The attitude a woman has to her body in general, and labour in particular, is likely to affect her interpretation of the new sensations called contractions. Women who come to labour with a positive attitude seem to need less analgesia,[5] as do women who reacted positively to the onset of menstruation. It is likely that a woman who does not regard new bodily sensations as automatically injurious or threatening will not prejudge the sensations of labour.

Women who have positive feelings towards their unborn baby and towards their partners also have better experiences of birth. As has been remarked, there seems a certain injustice in the fact that, where the experience of birth is concerned, to those who have it shall be given.[20] Thus a well-educated, mature, happily married woman of high socio-economic status who has attended antenatal classes, and who labours with her husband by her side, is more likely to enjoy her labour than a woman for whom these factors do not operate.[5, 6] Important though these statistics are in enabling health professionals to identify those women in most need of their help and support, with the exception of attendance at antenatal classes, they are not factors over which women have much control at the time they are contemplating labour. Of more interest to women in general are the factors which positively influence their perception of labour over which they *do* have some control.

Women who have confidence in themselves as prospective birth-givers, a positive and independent attitude to childbirth and who do not expect to need analgesia, seem to be more likely to have a satisfactory birth experience and use less analgesia than those for whom this is not the case.[2, 5] Some women acquire this attitude as a result of their general experience of life, from hearing positive accounts of birth from their own mothers, close female relatives or friends, or absorbing it from the general ethos of their culture.

Others may find that their approach to labour becomes more positive as a result of attending good antenatal classes. Investigative studies have repeatedly found that women who have attended antenatal classes have a more positive birth experience and use less analgesia than those who do not.[5, 6, 21, 22, 23] It has been suggested that the sort of woman who attends antenatal classes is quite likely to have a positive attitude (and probably a good education) already and that attitudes predispose women to take classes rather than classes altering attitude and outcome. This suggestion was examined in a survey which compared the outcome of women who wanted classes and took them, with women who wanted classes but could not take them because they were full.[24] It was also examined by other researchers[25, 26] who randomly assigned women to receive or not to receive classes, thereby avoiding the self-selection bias in another way. All three studies found statistically significant differences in the amount of analgesia used by the women who had received antenatal education when compared with those who had not. To use the earlier analogy, 'a clear understanding of the rules of the game and what is involved in playing' is likely to be helpful to a woman facing labour, whether she obtains this from her own mother, her midwife, her antenatal class, or failing all these, a good book, film or video. Much of the fear of labour is generated by simply not knowing what to expect and being unable to visualize the effect the perceived sensations are having.

> . . . I was soon into good contractions and floated over them with the shallowest breathing I've ever experienced. I didn't realize one could breathe like that, practising. It's quite true that practise simply gives you a theory and the experience pushes you into what you need . . .

As well as approaching labour well-informed, well-prepared and with a positive attitude, it is necessary to be aware of other, external factors which will influence the perception of labour and the experience of birth. These could be described as 'scene-setting', but they also may profoundly affect a woman's experience of birth.

Most other mammals have no need of care-givers or labour companions, so their primary occupation, when labour approaches is to find a quiet, safe, warm, comfortable, private environment for birth. Even for (uncaged) domestic animals, this will be a place of their own choosing, and owners may sometimes be quite put out to find that the nice cosy box they provided for the birth is not what the animal wants at all, and the litter is produced in the back of a wardrobe or behind the sofa.

Similarly, a woman cannot 'give herself over' to her labour if she is constantly aware that she might be interrupted, particularly by strangers. Her body's response to continual small surges of adrenalin may be unpredictable, but she cannot labour optimally under these conditions. (As Sheila Kitzinger has often said, 'the room where the baby is born should be the room in which it was or could have been conceived').

The environment for birth has received attention recently, and attempts have been made to make hospital settings more home-like; ranging from the addition of pretty wallpaper and curtains to furnishing the whole room as if it were a bedroom. This is undoubtedly a step in the right direction, for research in other areas has shown that in a hospital setting, a person's well-being can be influenced by their surroundings.[27]

However, 'the environment for birth' is more than just a matter of fixtures and fittings. It is also greatly affected by the attitudes, philosophies and personalities of the care-givers, by the system of care-giving and the place of birth itself.

> . . . The midwife was marvellous—she also watched my face and listened to me to find out how strong the contractions were. Incidentally everything was lovely and quiet all the time—I felt as if I was the only person giving birth in the hospital, which was as it should be . . .

In many cultures women labour with the companionship of other women, either relatives or friends, and birth is not regarded as something a woman could or should do on her own. Yet in societies that regard themselves as 'civilized' it is very often the case that women are left alone in labour. The damaging effects of 'isolating' a labouring woman from social support[28] have been clearly demonstrated[29], and many hospitals now accept (and even welcome) the presence of the labour companion(s) of the woman's choice. However not all women are in the situation of having someone who is willing and able to be with them throughout labour, and for these women it is particularly important that they are able to opt for the system of professional care that is most likely to ensure that they will receive constant support in labour from a midwife, preferably one that they have come to know and trust during their pregnancy.

> . . . The midwife stroked my arm, which I found comforting, and gave me sips of the water we'd brought in and lots of encouragement. Sometime around midnight she said I was nearly there and at about quarter past twelve her encouragement to push coincided with my inability to do anything else! At about this point my membranes popped with a ping and a warm gush—I was thrilled to have reached the second stage with the membranes intact . . .

It has been repeatedly shown that the system of care which gives mothers and midwives the greatest satisfaction, and is associated with a reduced need for analgesics in labour (by comparison with other systems of care), is that which enables women to get to know and receive care from a very small number of midwives during pregnancy, labour and the postnatal period.[30, 31] Continuity of care enables the woman and her midwife to see and respond to each other as individuals (and often as friends). This will make a difference clinically, as the midwife will always be able to compare 'this time' with 'last time' and subtle differences are less likely to go unnoticed. It will mean that the effects of any advice given can be seen and if necessary modified by the same person. More especially, in the context of labour, it will mean that the woman is not cared for by a stranger, or worse still, a succession of strangers.

Most women in Britain give birth in a hospital of some sort, and it is possible to achieve all that research (and mothers and midwives) regard as desirable in a hospital setting (see Chapters 3 and 4). But it may require a considerable expenditure of effort and energy on the part of a pregnant woman to try to ensure that when she finally goes into labour the people, the setting and the care are right for her. Few women regard with equanimity the prospect of receiving their antenatal care from a succession of strangers on their repeated visits to a hospital, or their care in labour from yet more strangers who may be constrained by hospital policy from treating them as individuals. They may dread the thought of receiving endless 'conflicting advice' in the vulnerable, early postnatal period. However in some areas it will be very difficult for them to negotiate the kind of care they want whilst 'booked' (often only nominally) with a consultant.

All women should be aware that there are alternatives to hospital as the place of birth (i.e. GP units and home) and to 'shared care' or consultant unit care (i.e. community-based midwifery care in a variety of forms); and that these are realistic options for (the majority of) women who are not specifically considered to be in need of specialist medical/obstetrical care. These alternatives will be discussed in more detail in Chapters 3 and 4.

Good information to reduce the fear of the unknown, appropriate muscle response to the sensations of labour, positive attitude, companionship in labour, continuity of care, ability to move freely in labour, privacy, warmth, quiet, emotional support, and the avoidance of interventive techniques such as the use of oxytocin and artificial rupture of the membranes to induce or augment labour (in the absence of specific indications) are all factors associated with a reduced need for analgesia and therefore (presumably) an increased ability to cope with labour: Some of these factors are directly in the hands of the woman herself, but others are more or less likely to operate in the case of an individual woman according to the choices she makes about where she will have her baby and who will provide her care. Every woman will make these decisions at some level, even if her decision is to let someone else decide. What she will face, in every case, are the consequences of those decisions.

3 Attitudes to Pregnancy and Birth

It may be regarded as an oversimplification, but in general people take up one of two possible positions with regard to the process of childbirth; either it is a physiological process that can be regarded as normal until it has been shown (in an individual case) to be otherwise, or else it is only normal in retrospect. (Analogous in law to a person being regarded as innocent until proved guilty, or guilty until proved innocent.)

The ability to reproduce and to metabolize are the two fundamental properties of all living things, from the simplest microorganism upwards. On a higher evolutionary level, these two processes subdivide into the eight physiological characteristics of the animal kingdom. All animals have the ability to move, feed, breathe, excrete, circulate blood, co-ordinate their functioning by means of a nervous system, exhibit instinctive and often learnt behaviour, and to reproduce.[1] All these are regarded as normal, physiological functions. That is not to say that they never go wrong or develop faults — indeed many medical textbooks have chapters headed 'diseases of the respiratory system', 'diseases of the digestive system' or 'diseases of the cardiovascular system'. But no-one suggests that breathing or eating are in themselves diseases or illnesses, or even, despite the fact that Britain has the highest incidence of cardiovascular disease in the world, (after Sweden), that everyone should be equipped with a defibrillator and a respirator, 'just in case'.

Yet paradoxically over the course of the last century, as the death of either a mother or baby in childbirth has become rarer and rarer, the reproductive process has increasingly come to be regarded as pathological. This state of affairs seems to have arisen from a combination of many factors, amongst which must be the increase in the number of hospital confinements, thus taking birth out of the mainstream of life and making it mysterious; and the increasing involvement of doctors in the care of childbearing women.

Historically the move towards increased hospital confinement had very little to do with safety. The first national analysis of the place of delivery in England and Wales appeared in the Registrar General's statistical review of 1927, which reported that only 15 per cent of births took place in institutions of some sort, ranging from workhouses to lying-in hospitals. Five years later, his second report noted an increase in institutional deliveries and ascribed these largely to economic changes — more people were receiving poor relief and institutionalized deliveries were cheaper.[2]

More seriously the report also noted that there had been a rise in maternal mortality from obstetric intervention. This had arisen partly because midwives attending difficult births were now obliged (by the medically inspired 1902 Midwives Act) to send for a doctor, who in some cases would have had inadequate training and experience; and partly because middle class women were more likely to be able to pay to be attended by doctors rather than midwives, thereby putting themselves at increased risk of unwarranted and sometimes inexpert intervention.[3]

A significant factor in the further rise in institutionalized births was the Second World War, when, because of the danger from air raids, pregnant women in inner city areas were evacuated to emergency medical service hospitals. Thus by the end of the war 'hospital' had become the focus for birth. This was maintained, according to the Chief Medical Officer's Report of 1952, partly because it became a free service after 1948, and partly because at a time of high employment there were fewer female relatives on hand to help with home births.

Then in 1959 came the Cranbrook Report which suggested, without any supporting statistics, that seventy per cent was the optimum percentage of births that should take place in hospital. This was followed by the Peel Report in 1970 which suggested that this percentage should be raised to 100 per cent. It is conceivable that this recommendation had been influenced more by the under-utilization of hospital beds that had been provided in response to the 'post war bulge' (and which were now lying empty as the birth rate fell again) than by concern for health, because this report again failed to provide any statistical support for its claims of greater safety in institutions.[2]

Thus it would appear that financial constraints played a much greater part than safety in channelling women towards hospital confinements; but given that hospitals were and are places where the sick are treated, it is not surprising that the link has been made, in some minds, between pregnancy and sickness. This connection has been strengthened by the increasing involvement of doctors in pregnancy care.

The philosophical basis of modern medicine, as with other branches of science, was laid by Descartes, who argued that the path to truth lay only in those things that could be known by adopting a logical, quantitative, reductionist approach.[4] In medicine this resulted in a mechanistic, objective view of the human body, with the emphasis on curative rather than preventative care. This view of bio-social human experiences such as health, birth and death makes them 'manageable', but it also makes them pathological because they are seen purely negatively, in terms of problems and solutions.[5] This problem-oriented view of health means that, for most doctors, the vast majority of the population divides into those who are 'not sick', who they don't see, and those who are sick, who they treat.

This pathological perception of health is reinforced by a predominantly hospital-based training, during which time, as the medical student progresses towards his/her ultimate goal, s/he learns to cope with sick people, who want pain relief, nursing care, relief from responsibility and a cure for their illness. To meet their needs s/he becomes authoritarian, didactic and all-knowing.[6]

In the fullness of time, some of these doctors become obstetricians. Others have speculated on the reasons why men might choose to become obstetricians,[6] but even more important than their reasons is the effect that their prior training and orientation have on childbearing women. The reductionist approach to pregnancy care considers individual practices and interventions in isolation, without considering their implications. For example, every European country, according to the World Health Organization's regional officer for maternal and child health, has a different concept of what constitutes 'risk' in pregnancy, largely because there is no firm evidence on which to base such concepts. The only thing which the many screening tests that are set up have in common is a high 'false positive' rate, which results in a great number of women being erroneously labelled 'high risk'; as many as fifty per cent in some countries.[5, 7]

In this country an examination of the case records of all the women delivering in Aberdeen in one year (1975) found that of 289 women whose babies were diagnosed as suffering from intra-uterine growth retardation (i.e. they appeared to be smaller than they should have been for a particular period of pregnancy), only 83 were confirmed at birth — 2.5 false positives for every case correctly identified.[8]

High-risk women are more likely to have their labours induced, and induced labours are more likely to require pharmacological pain relief,[9] the use of which increases the likelihood of an operative delivery.[10] Women deemed to be at high risk are also more likely to have their labours monitored electronically, a technique which has been shown repeatedly to increase the incidence of caesarean section.[11] Thus among the consequences of this reductionist approach may be an epidemic of neonatal intensive care and self-fulfilling prophecies.

The attitude to childbirth which leads to so many women being regarded as 'high risk' also affects the type of care given to those who are 'officially' low risk. Care-givers who are so suspicious of (or have so little respect for) the birth process that they are 'waiting for something to go wrong' are far more likely to intervene in normal labour than those to whom labour is essentially a normal physiological function. Since it is very difficult to perform any procedure during labour in isolation, many 'low-risk' women find themselves caught up in the 'cascade of intervention'[12] as a result.

The reductionist approach to birth also has an effect on the health care structure itself. The sort of technology that has been developed, e.g. ultrasound scanning, requires that women go to where the technology is, and antenatal care is thus moved from a community base to a hospital base. This has all sorts of socio-economic repercussions, which ultimately mean that the women most in need of pregnancy care are least likely to get it.

Modern technology also affects the training and skills of the people giving the care. Eyes, hands and ears are being devalued and skills are being lost. If the care giver always uses a sonicaid to listen to the baby's heart rate, s/he will lose the ability to hear it just with an ear; if s/he relies on a monitor to give information about the strength and frequency of a woman's contractions, s/he will lose the ability to detect it with just a hand (or by talking to the woman). Obstetricians who work in hospitals where all breech births are routinely delivered by caesarean section will feel alarmed at the prospect of a vaginal breech delivery; and more and more midwives feel too insecure to attend home deliveries because they have seen so few.

As well as having a significant effect on the health care structure, a negative, problem-oriented view of birth will have a profound effect on the individual pregnant woman. A woman pregnant for the first time is undergoing a major life experience. There are few things that so radically change a woman's perceptions, attitudes, relationships and priorities than the birth of her first child. The most important of these is her changing view of herself. She has to move from being someone's daughter to being someone's mother. Compared with the time for which she has been someone's daughter, nine months is not very long for this maturation to take place, and the process of learning to take responsibility for herself and her child needs to be cultivated from the very beginning. In women who appear ready and willing to take it, it needs to be encouraged, in those who are not it needs to be developed.

But to do this the pregnant women will need rather different attitudes and skills from those which the obstetrician with a conventional medical background has been trained to provide. The doctor's response to the sick person, that of curing, reassuring authoritarianism, is of little use to a woman who wants information, autonomy, support and to share decision-making. Unfortunately few doctors yet learn how to be permissive, nondirective counsellors, with the result that they often react very defensively to demands which seem to challenge their judgment and expertise. (Many obstetricians are unable to see that part of the reason for the 'demands' which are a thorn in the flesh of so many of them, is that their entrenched medical orientation makes it very difficult for women to 'ask' for something, without seeming to be fighting and demanding it.)[8] Yet it is an essential part of the psychological transition to motherhood that women persuade professionals to stop regarding them as 'sick' and therefore child-like and to share with them the responsibility for their care.

4 Care during Pregnancy and Birth

One of the first things a woman is likely to do when she realizes that she is pregnant, is to go and see her doctor. (When the word 'midwife' in this first sentence can be substituted for the word 'doctor', most of the rest of this chapter will have become unnecessary!)

At that first visit, particularly if this is her first pregnancy, the main thing on her mind will probably be the impact that 'being pregnant' is going to have on her life, and how she will cope with it. It is rather less likely that she will be aware that decisions are being made that will affect not only how and where she gives birth and the type of care she receives during her pregnancy, labour and postnatal period; but also the ease with which future choices can be made, for example over labour procedures, behaviour in labour or who is present at delivery.

A prerequisite of real choice is that there is a comprehensive set of options, and that the chooser has the power to exercise that choice freely and in an informed way, with the proviso that the rights of others are neither ignored nor infringed.[1,2] Choice, when exercised in this way, tends to promote responsibility; and mothers (and fathers) should have the right to take responsibility for their own health and that of their children, if for no other reason than that it is they who will have to cope, in the short and long term, with the consequences of decisions taken during pregnancy or at the time of birth.

For most pregnant women, this visit is their first encounter with a professional 'attitude' to childbirth, even though this is not always apparent. If the woman is to be 'booked' for delivery at this visit, she should be made aware that there are potentially four options open to her; she could have her baby in a consultant unit, in a GP unit within a larger maternity unit, in an outlying GP unit, or in her own home. If she has not considered these options before, she should be given an opportunity to discuss their implications, both with her doctor and with anyone else she feels should be consulted. This is a time-consuming operation for busy professionals, particularly if they are already convinced in their own mind what the best course of action should be, but anything less is not 'informed choice', it is 'Hobson's choice'.

Furthermore, those GPs who do not practice obstetrics and automatically book their pregnant 'patients' for hospital deliveries, and those who do practise obstetrics but automatically book all first-time mothers for hospital delivery without discussion, are making a basic (and automatic) assumption about the safety and desirability of a hospital confinement which the evidence suggests that they are not entitled to make.[3] It is highly unlikely that the majority of GPs who do this are deliberately trying to deceive women, but they have been told for so long that hospital delivery is safer that it is not surprising that they believe it.

There will always be a small proportion of the pregnant population who need the particular type of care that only consultant units can provide, and it could not be argued that these women would be better off at home or in GP units. Nevertheless it has been repeatedly demonstrated that, for the vast majority, hospital delivery is not safer than delivery in GP units or at home. Tew came to this conclusion after analyzing *national* perinatal morality statistics.[4] (The perinatal mortality rate, the number of babies either born dead or dying within the first week of birth, per 1000 total births, is a crude, if unambiguous measurement of 'success' in obstetrics.) Others have come to similar conclusions by analyzing data for different regions in this and other countries.

A GP in Newcastle-upon-Tyne looked at the outcome of 701 consecutive pregnant women on one GP's list, over a 15-year period (from 1962–1976). Seventy per cent of these women had delivered in the GP unit, and the average perinatal mortality rate for these women was less than half that of both the national and the area average.[5] Another doctor in Reading compared the outcomes, in terms of perinatal mortality, of 1686 women delivered in the GP units in Henley, Newbury, Reading and Wokingham, with 1271 women who met the well-defined GP unit booking criteria of the West Berkshire GP units, but who were delivered in Rochdale and the Isle of Wight where there were no GP units. He found no difference in the perinatal morality rates between the two groups, and suggested that this cast serious doubt on the argument that booking all women in consultant units would solve the problem of the acknowledged higher perinatal mortality rates amongst infants whose mothers were transferred from GP unit to consultant care.[6]

In 1982 a community physician in Oxfordshire, compared the perinatal mortality rates in Oxford, where at that time 12 per cent of deliveries took place in the GP unit, with those in Banbury, where 45 per cent of deliveries took place in the GP unit. He concluded that there was no difference in the two rates for babies who weighed over 2500 gm, and only slight, but statistically insignificant differences for babies of lower birth weights.[7]

Moving further afield, a survey determined the perinatal mortality rates for all the public hospitals in New Zealand between 1978 and 1981. About 40 per cent of all births took place in small rural units staffed by GPs and midwives, and the other 60 per cent in either regional hospitals or in the few major referral centres. It found that for the 94 per cent of births in which the babies were of normal birth weight, the perinatal mortality rate was significantly lower in the smaller units. Furthermore there was no evidence that satisfactory outcome was dependent on a minimum number of deliveries per year — an argument that is often used by those who regard the closure of small GP units as desirable. On the contrary, the perinatal mortality rates were lowest in units with less than 100 deliveries per year, and highest in those with more than 2000 deliveries per year.[8]

Returning to this country, another survey of all 8856 births that had taken place at home in England and Wales in 1979 looked at the outcome of the birth in relation to the *intended* place of delivery, not the *actual* place of delivery.[9] In other words, if the baby was due to be born at home, but the mother needed to be transferred to hospital during labour, with the result that the baby was actually born in hospital, it was counted as an 'intended home birth'. Similarly, a birth that was planned to take place in hospital, but for some reason took place at home, was counted as an 'intended hospital birth'.

It was found that if the home birth had been booked for delivery at home (as opposed to being an unplanned home delivery), the perinatal mortality rate was very low; 4.1 per 1000, at a time when the national average was 14.7 per 1000. It also showed quite clearly that 30 per cent of the births that had taken place at home had actually been booked for hospital, or not booked at all (e.g. a concealed pregnancy). These births had a perinatal mortality rate of 67.5 per 1000, and 30 per cent of the babies were of low birth weight. The study had been undertaken in response to the Short Committee's recommendation that home births should be phased out further, which had been made because they had accepted at face value the fact that by 1977 the perinatal mortality rate for all home births was higher than that for consultant units. As a result of the study it became clear that 'all home births' included a large number of high-risk, unplanned home births, which ought not to have been included in discussions about the desirability of planned home births. The findings also provided a counter-argument to those who suggest that if women could be dissuaded from giving birth at home, there would be no need to maintain flying squad facilities. It became apparent that it was the high-risk, unplanned home birth group that was most likely to need its services, not the low-risk planned group.

Two senior academics have recently reviewed research studies from all over the world,[10] in which low-technology midwife/GP care was compared with high-technology specialist care. They were surprised to find that in every study the outcomes for mothers and babies were better in the midwife/GP group than in the specialist group; the only exception to this was in the case of babies of very low birth weight.

What most obstetricians have meant in the past when they have maintained that hospital delivery is safer, is that a woman, and more particularly a child, are less likely to die if delivered there than elsewhere. Not only is it becoming increasingly obvious that this is not true, it also ignores the fact that, as has often been said, there is a great deal more to being alive than simply not being dead. At the moment there is no national maternal or perinatal morbidity equivalent to the three-yearly audit published as Confidential Enquiries into Maternal Deaths. A reporting system of this type has now been called for by two anaesthetists.[11] But even so, it is envisaged as a register for fairly major events, resulting in physical damage. There are other sorts of morbidity which are so common that the mother may be regarded as 'well' by the traditional criteria for successful obstetric management; episiotomy, for example.

It is also difficult to see how the objective world of obstetric concern would classify the psychological damage done to a woman, which can have repercussions beyond the immediate postnatal period. She may be regarded as perfectly normal obstetrically and yet have been 'deeply disturbed and humiliated to more than a temporary degree by her experience'.[12]

Differences in morbidity between specialist care and midwife/GP care in labour for women and their babies at similar pre-delivery risk have been well illustrated by a number of studies. A Californian study compared 500 births that took place in an alternative birthing room (ABR) and received midwifery care, with 500 that took place in a conventional delivery room (CDR).[13] All the women were assessed as being at similarly low pre-delivery risk. The women in the ABR had no intravenous fluids or electronic fetal monitoring as a matter of routine. They were allowed to adopt whatever posture they liked and have their families with them if they so desired. Only 6 per cent of these women had up to 75 mg of pethidine (a pain-killer) during labour.

In contrast, all the women in the CDR (which was actually next door!) had intravenous fluids, 81 per cent of them had electronic fetal monitoring, 29 per cent had epidurals and 69 per cent had at least 75 mg of pethidine. Statistically significant differences were seen between the two groups in the number who failed to progress in labour (18.3 per cent CDR; 5.2 per cent ABR), received oxytocin (21 per cent CDR; 3.1 per cent

ABR), had fetal distress diagnosed (5.3 per cent CDR; 0.3 per cent ABR), had meconium-stained amniotic fluid (11.9 per cent CDR; 2.3 per cent ABR) and had caesarean sections (9.2 per cent CDR; 2.8 per cent ABR). Among the babies significant differences were found in the incidence of jaundice (12.6 per cent CDR; 2.4 per cent ABR) and scalp infections (1.2 per cent CDR; 0 per cent ABR).

Four years previously, similar differences were found between the outcomes of 1046 home and 1046 hospital births, which were all at similar pre-delivery risk. The women delivered in hospital had a much greater incidence of forceps deliveries, caesarean sections, labour induction and augmentation with oxytocin; vastly more episiotomies and yet also more serious perineal tears; more actively managed third stages and yet more incidents of serious bleeding after birth; and more babies with birth injuries, infections and other non-congenital complications.[14].

In this country, similar comparisons have been made between two groups of 126 low-risk women, who delivered either in a consultant unit or a GP unit within the same (!) larger maternity unit. Although the labour rooms were identical and all facilities were equally available to both groups, the 'systems of care' were quite different. In one group, women were booked for the consultant unit, and their antenatal care was 'shared' between their GP and the hospital antenatal clinic. Although they may have known their GP quite well they would have been very unlikely to have seen anyone they knew on any of the trips they made to the antenatal clinic, just whoever was on duty that day. It is quite probable that they never saw the consultant whose name appeared on their case notes. Even if they had seen any of the clinic midwives on more than one occasion, it would be very unlikely that they would have met them again in the delivery suite (student midwives and internal rotation notwithstanding), as all the staff in individual departments of the hospital are effectively separate. They would have seen yet more strangers on the postnatal wards after their delivery.

The women who were booked for the GP unit, on the other hand, would have received their care from their GP, whom they might already know, and their 'own' midwife and her three colleagues, whom they would have had the opportunity, throughout their pregnancies, of getting to know. This continuity would have continued throughout their labour and postnatal care as well.

The comparison began at the point at which the woman contacted her midwife or the hospital because she believed herself to be in labour; thus women who had labour induced were excluded.

The study found that the women in the shared care group had significantly more interventions; more augmentation of labour, more electronic fetal monitoring, more analgesia, more anaesthesia, more epidurals and more forceps deliveries. Their babies were also more likely to have fetal distress diagnosed and to require intubation (to help them breathe in the first few minutes after birth).[15]

In the only prospective, randomized controlled trial to assess the impact of these two types of care on the women who receive them, 1000 low-risk women attending St George's Hospital in London were assigned randomly (with their consent) to two groups. The experimental group received nearly all their antenatal, labour and postnatal care from a team of four midwives (the Know Your Midwife group) while the other group received the conventional fragmented hospital care. The groups were compared in terms of feasibility, satisfaction, obstetric outcome and cost. The women who received their care from midwives they knew were more satisfied with their antenatal care, saw fewer professionals, had fewer antenatal hospital admissions, felt better prepared for labour, felt more in control during labour and had a more positive experience of labour than those in the control group. They had less intervention, less analgesia, fewer epidurals and more normal deliveries. (Midwife care was also found to be cheaper, for a variety of reasons.)[16]

The conclusion that can be drawn from these studies is once again that low-risk women and their babies (the majority of the population) fare better if given low-technology, personalized care.

However, not all women are swayed by research evidence, (any more than all obstetricians and midwives seem to be). Women have been told so often and in so many ways that hospital is safe and anywhere else is dangerous that it is hardly surprising that most of them believe it. That being the case it would be just as unreasonable to compel women with no antici-pated need for hospital facilities to give birth at home as it is to insist that they go to a hospital. In all labours peace of mind is an important factor, and women should be able to give birth in the place where they feel safe and secure — which for a pro-portion will mean hospital. There are some women who cope with labour by handing over responsibility to others; they want their labours managed and controlled, and, in general, their needs are well-catered for by the average consultant/obstetric unit.

There are others, a majority perhaps, who wish to remain an active participant in the process of giving birth. This is the group who are often badly served in hospital consultant units. Too much of their energy and attention is used up trying to ward off unnecessary intervention, and striving to maintain the personal uniqueness of their own pregnancy and labour. The consequence of their failure in this respect was made apparent, yet again, by the accounts of two mothers who were addressing a large, multidisciplinary gathering of health care professionals at a recent meeting at the Royal Society of Medicine's Forum on Maternity and the Newborn. They described in detail their tremendous sense of loss, particularly of self-respect and self control.

One of them said that during the course of her first labour she had felt part of herself 'slipping away'. Her inability to reconcile the person she had been before her labour with the person she now thought that she was, resulted in two years of depression. The other mother described her overwhelming sense of failure which had left her feeling that there was a personal battle that she had to win in order to restore her lost self-esteem. Her emotional reaction to her fundamental loss of autonomy in her labour had, she maintained, governed her early relationship with her child.[17]

Both of these mothers were saying what any mother will say; that birth is a major and unique event that is remembered for a lifetime; and it is not *just* a matter of a healthy mother and child, as the thousands of letters that AIMS (the Association for

Improvements in the Maternity Services) receive every year will testify. (What ultimately restored the self-esteem of these two women was the care that they had received in their most recent pregnancy, during which time they had been able to establish a relationship of trust with their midwife and retain their autonomy in labour.)

Women's experiences and opinions are necessarily subjective and cannot be quantified in the same way as physiological or technological events. For this reason they are frequently dismissed as being of no clinical interest; 'a side-line, perhaps, for individual liberal obstetricians to interest themselves in, but marginal to the real work'.[12] The only possible device for endowing these subjective experiences with objectivity is to amass a series of accounts of individual experiences and extrapolate from these,[18] as Sheila Kitzinger, among others, regularly and effectively does.[19, 20]

One of the reasons why women's feelings can be totally disregarded in a hospital setting is that the power relationships between the givers and receivers of care, both in pregnancy and labour, are often very unequal. Once most prospective parents enter a hospital they become relatively powerless; and at the heart of this is the lack of opportunity to form a personal or social relationship.

This stems largely from the fact that 'hospitals are large and complex social institutions in which staff are organized hierarchically and relationships are predominantly bureaucratic. That is to say, relations among staff, and between staff and the people for whom they care, are based on such things as status and role and not on the more personal and spontaneous factors that characterize relationships in the less public spheres of life. Bureaucratic institutions are specifically designed so that one individual can be replaced by another who can perform the same function'.[21] Rule-following and the avoidance of responsibility are typical of large institutions. (This has its ultimate expression in the National Maternity Hospital in Dublin, the heart of active management, where, provided the rules are followed precisely, the Master takes full responsibility for the actions of his subordinates.) This of course has profound implications for the quality of the relationships that are possible, as each attendant comes and goes in a series of brief encounters. Human beings are social animals and gain their sense of individual identity and worth from their relationships with others. They can thus be just as effectively isolated in a crowd of strangers as in an empty room. Their sense of powerlessness in hospital is reinforced by an awareness of being on someone else's territory, and they are consequently under strong pressure, both direct and indirect, to accept hospital routines and submit to their (often ritualistic) procedures.

The question 'What do women want?' is meaningless because women vary, and therefore want different things; 'They do not exist "en bloc" as a category of people whose needs can be met by a single piece of mass legislation'.[12] Hence again the need for choice. However it often appears to be the case that 'some people have a subconscious idea that women are an altogether less complex species, more like, shall we say, rhododendrons or beans, so that somewhere, just around the corner, is a simple answer on the lines of "They need plenty of phosphates" and that once this secret has been discovered life will be simpler. Women can be given what they want and they will then keep quiet, thus enabling the time and attention of real (i.e. male) people to be devoted to the important and difficult business of conducting their relationships with other real people.'[22] The same writer goes on to say; 'This concept, like the concept of the oral aphrodisiac, is a male mirage; such a formula will never be found. All we can do is to try and disentangle some of the factors contributing to the discontent of women at the present time.'

What the women at the Royal Society of Medicine said they wanted, in common with many of the women who have written to AIMS, and no doubt many who have not, was a personal, continuous relationship with their midwife throughout pregnancy, labour and the postnatal period, so that they had the opportunity and the time to establish a relationship of trust. They wanted privacy, a relaxed and optimistic attitude to the process of labour; support, encouragement and explanation.

All these things come almost automatically if the woman and her midwife can establish a personal continuing, social relationship. This is not impossible, even in a hospital setting, as Caroline Flint has so ably demonstrated,[16] but it requires a basic re-organization of the established structure.

It has been argued that in the case of maternity care, even if it is only a minority of women who express a particular unmet need or disappointment, they cannot be dismissed simply because they are a minority. 'The paradigm is not that of a vote in parliamentary election, where only one candidate can get in. A situation which involves a response to the social, cultural, psychological and medical needs of 50 per cent of the population calls for flexibility and a series of possible choices . . . (If only a few women object to remaining flat on their backs during delivery, but it is also clear that this is an inefficient position, then there is every reason to offer everyone alternative and better positions, regardless of the fact that in the first place, only a minority complained.) Flexibility may also be cheaper too,[16] although this is not a final argument.'[12]

Slowly, efforts are being made to introduce 'team midwifery' schemes for women who would otherwise be offered the conventional, fragmented, 'consultant' care, but for most women this is not yet an option.

For the majority of women, the four potential options discussed at the beginning of this chapter are the ones they should be given the opportunity to consider. Each woman's first consideration should be whether there is anything in her medical, obstetric (or even social) history, or any aspect of her current pregnancy, that warrants specialized care from, or delivery in, a consultant obstetric unit. Most places have well-defined criteria for what constitutes 'high' and 'low' risk in the context of making an initial decision about the type of care and the place of birth. Some of these criteria are negotiable and are often a good place to start (see Appendix 1). Ultimately the individual woman has the power of veto, whether she uses it or not.

A hospital booking will involve some or all of her antenatal care being given at the hospital (often it will be shared with her GP). She is unlikely to meet the same person twice in a hospital antenatal clinic. She will be cared for in labour by midwives she has never met, and may encounter several shifts of midwives if her labour is longer than 8 hours.

After the birth, if she remains in the hospital, she will be cared for by yet more midwives that she has never met, working in shifts, and finally, when she goes home, she will receive her care from the community-based (often part-time) midwives, whom she may conceivably have met antenatally, but will more probably be strangers to her. The quality of care she receives may be excellent; it may be tailored to her individual needs; or it may not.

A GP unit booking will require first of all that she is registered to receive maternity care with a GP who is on the 'obstetric list' (as held by the Family Practitioner Committee — 'FPC') and who uses the local GP unit, if there is one. Sometimes the GP with whom the woman is currently registered also does GP obstetrics, sometimes it will be necessary for her to register, temporarily, with another, just for maternity care, without leaving her own GP's list.

For the name of a suitable GP, she could ask the FPC, the head of the local community midwifery service, the local branch of the NCT (National Childbirth Trust), or her friends.

She will then be assigned to a particular midwife, who will come to see her at home, and together they will fill in her notes, which in many cases she will then be given to keep during the pregnancy. More particularly, the foundation of an on-going relationship will be laid that will continue throughout pregnancy, labour and the postnatal period, and may often develop into a long-term friendship.

During the course of her pregnancy the mother should also meet the other (usually three) members of 'her' midwife's group or team, from whom she may receive some of her care. Thus in labour she will be cared for by someone she knows.

The actual birth will take place wherever the GP unit is, either within a large maternity unit, or some distance from it.

Essentially the same system of care will operate, in most cases, if a woman decides to have her baby at home; i.e. she will be cared for by her midwife and her team, in conjunction with her GP.

However, a woman is under no legal obligation to have the services of a doctor, and if she is unable to find one willing to accept her for a home delivery, she can obtain the services of a midwife on her own, either privately, or through the local community midwifery service. The services of the NHS mid-wife are obtained by contacting the Director of Midwifery Services, or if there is one, the Senior Midwife for Community Midwifery (see Appendix 2). The midwife provided (and the Health Authority have a duty to provide one) will be acting as a practitioner in her own right, and will be responsible for all the woman's care. Even if the midwife feels it is inadvisable for the woman to be delivered at home, she still has a duty (unless she is relieved and replaced) to continue her attendance on the mother. It is up to the midwife, not the woman, to arrange medical/obstetric cover in case it is needed.

No woman can avoid taking risks in her decision-making, any more than any other adult can, and in most areas of life this is taken for granted. Every time a road is crossed, a gas stove is lit or an aeroplane takes off, someone is taking a calculated risk. Deciding to embark on a pregnancy involves taking a calculated risk, so too does deciding where to give birth. Furthermore, no woman can, in any real sense, avoid making this decision. If she decides to 'leave everything to you, Doctor' she has made a decision, and taken a risk. If she allows herself to be confined in hospital, without discussing the reasons for it, she is taking the risk that her advisors may not be considering her individual needs but merely following policy (government, regional, or district); and that once in hospital, the risks of unnecessary interference, lack of continuity of care etc. are not greater than the potential benefits conferred on her by being there. If she consciously makes a choice, whatever that choice is, she must have judged for herself that on balance, and in her circumstances, the potential benefits of her chosen place of confinement appear to outweigh the potential hazards. All that professionals and others can do is to make sure that the woman has as much accurate information as she wants so that she can make an informed choice.

5 Preparing for Labour

Labour 'preparation' could be considered in two halves; half is the individual woman preparing herself, physically, mentally and practically for the process of labour, and the other half is ensuring that the system of care and the prospective environment for labour will come as close to meeting her individual needs as she can manage.

The first step, as became apparent in Chapter 4, is to consider the four 'place of birth' options, and their accompanying systems of care. For the sake of completeness, a fifth system should be mentioned; the Domino (DOMiciliary-IN-and Out) delivery. Here the local community midwife books the woman and sees her throughout her pregnancy, usually at her GP's clinic. When she goes into labour, the woman calls the midwife who attends her in her home until labour is well established, at which point they both move to the hospital consultant unit for the delivery. After the birth, if all is well, the woman rests in hospital for 6–24 hours and is transferred back home to the care of her midwife again. This system can work well, but it has drawbacks. Some hospitals do not 'allow' community midwives to stay on call for the women they have got to know in pregnancy, so women may end up by being delivered by a total stranger, which defeats the whole object of the exercise. Getting home from hospital sometimes causes problems if the Health Authority insist that women travel by ambulance, as long waits are often the result. Domino deliveries were once thought to be the ideal compromise, particularly in areas where there was no GP unit, for women who might otherwise have requested a home birth, but they do not seem to have met, nationally, with great success.[1,2]

The earlier in pregnancy these options are considered, the better, but it is perfectly possible for a woman who had been booked for a hospital delivery, only because she had not known that there were alternatives, to change her mind at a later date, provided she still has enough time left before the impending birth to make other arrangements. Similarly, women can change consultants within a hospital (most easily by talking to their GP) if they discover that 'their' consultant's policies conflict with their own preferences. They can also change their midwife, (by talking to her superior) in the event of a personality clash.

In the same way, a woman who was originally booked for a home or a GP unit delivery can be referred for a 'consultant opinion' or to 'consultant care' if difficulties arise in the pregnancy or in labour.

Whatever system of care a woman opts for, unless she plans to give birth at home she would be well advised to visit the place where she intends to have her baby. Not just the antenatal clinic, but the delivery area, special care nursery (if there is one) and the postnatal wards. Many hospitals offer 'guided tours' to expectant parents, and small groups are taken round by a member of staff, or, very occasionally, by the local NCT teacher. These tour leaders should be able to answer any questions that parents may have about the care given in the hospital. It may even be useful to make more than one tour, to gain a more rounded impression of what is available. It may also help a woman if the image of the room in which she will labour remains clearly in her mind, so that she can begin to picture herself there as she prepares for labour.

A few women who plan and anticipate a home birth may find themselves in hospital as a result of unforeseen difficulties, and it might thus be advisable for all women, regardless of where they plan to deliver, to go and see what their local hospital/GP unit looks like. Going in haste, in labour, to a place that she has imagined wrongly, is an additional stress that an antenatal tour of inspection could help to alleviate.

Few women would choose to labour alone, yet it is not

uncommon for labouring women to be left unattended for long periods in a hospital setting. The fact that this may be for reasons quite beyond the control of those responsible for the woman's care (shortage of staff, a sudden influx of women in labour) is no consolation to the individual woman. For this reason, among many others, it might be advisable for all pregnant women to arrange to have a companion with them in labour. The obvious choice is the baby's father, but not all men are comfortable with the prospect of being present during labour and birth, and a reluctant companion may be worse than no companion at all. Fear, embarrassment, distaste and other negative emotions emanating from anyone present during labour are counter-productive to the creation of an atmosphere of calm optimism, the optimum environment for labour. Labour companions can be drawn from among the woman's own female relatives or friends. Sometimes the woman will have an antenatal teacher, yoga teacher, acupuncturist etc. who is the most appropriate, willing companion.

A labour companion may do nothing throughout the course of the labour, sometimes just their presence is enough. On other occasions they may provide verbal and/or non-verbal forms of encouragement, appropriate massage, physical support, or drinks and cool flannels.

> . . . Towards the end of the first stage I did get amazingly irritated by small things; I remember even being cross with Tom for resting the newspaper across my legs . . . I sat cross-legged on a bed pan for a while rocking back and forth while Tom rubbed my back vigorously. It really is hard work . . . At about 10.15 I was offered some pethidine but refused it, feeling myself to be in good control albeit highly uncomfortable at the height of a contraction. Just before the incredible urge to push came I did threaten to turn into a whimpering heap, but that was where Tom was so marvellous, because he could see what was happening and give me instructions . . .

Because he or she is there exclusively in the interests of the labouring woman, a labour companion can act as an intermediary between the woman and her professional care-givers. He or she can forestall 'outside' distractions in the middle of contractions, provide professionals with a more detailed explanation of the woman's point of view than she is capable of giving herself while in labour, and repeat explanations if the woman is subject to any 'changes of shift'.

A labour companion may also suggest that the woman try out some of the options available to her, if such suggestions have not been made by anyone else. Given the right environment, many women will experiment quite unselfconsciously with different positions, cushions, waterbaths, showers, birthstools, etc. to increase their comfort. Others may need positive suggestions before they feel able to respond appropriately (see page 50).

In a situation where the woman has not had the opportunity of getting to know those caring for her in labour, her labour companion will be the only one present to whom she is known as a person, and in whom she can trust. It is remarkable how quickly a sense of rapport can develop between a labouring woman and a caring midwife whom she has not previously met, and midwives who are able to do this are often remembered with affection and gratitude for years after the event. However most women would probably prefer that such a relationship was not left to chance.

Most pregnant women will be asked, as part of the 'booking' procedure, if they intend to go to antenatal classes, and this is probably the most important way in which women can prepare themselves for labour and parenthood, regardless of their occupation or social situation.

Antenatal classes vary enormously in their content and usefulness, depending on where and by whom they are run. They may be run by the maternity hospital, by the local health centre, the National Childbirth Trust or a Birth Centre. The person teaching the course may be a midwife, health visitor, or a childbirth educator trained by a lay organization, e.g. NCT, Active Birth Centre. Some classes have general practitioners, obstetricians, midwives, breast-feeding counsellors and postnatal support group workers participating, and this may apply equally to NHS classes as to NCT/Birth Centre classes.

There are some significant differences between NHS classes

and those provided by lay organizations. NHS classes are free, take place on NHS property, are often composed of large numbers of people, may be led by different people on different weeks, and often cover a much wider range of subjects (often in a shorter period of time) than would be the case in, for example, NCT classes. Thus in addition to preparation for labour, such classes may cover diet, layette, baby care (bathing, nappy changing etc.), bottle-feeding demonstrations, immunizations and other aspects of a child's first year of life. In contrast, classes run by the National Childbirth Trust are usually held in the teacher's own home and consist of small groups, a maximum of eight women per group. This means that it is easy for each woman to get to know the other members of the group and for the teacher to get to know her. In this environment women can learn from each other and are less likely to feel constrained from asking questions through fear of being thought 'silly'. Although the teacher may invite others to contribute to part of certain classes, e.g. midwife, breast-feeding counsellor, she is always present and provides continuity from class to class. The other main difference is that most of the course is concerned with preparation for labour, physically and emotionally. Breast-feeding and the emotional aspects of early parenthood are also likely to be covered, but parentcraft is not. A small charge is made for NCT classes, although this can be reduced or waived if the woman would have difficulty paying.

There is no reason why a woman should not attend both sorts of classes if she wishes.

The depth to which each aspect of antenatal preparation is covered in a course of antenatal classes depends on several factors; who is teaching the class, whether the same person teaches on each occasion, and the time that can be allocated to each aspect. A course that has time to deal in depth with preparation for labour might include some or all of the following:

1. Information-giving, or information-sharing, depending on the background of the individual participants. This would include basic anatomy and physiology, an outline of the course of the three stages of labour, how a baby is normally born, variations from normal, common hospital procedures,

etc. (It will be necessary to point out that 'average' is only a concept, and that the labours of most of the women in the class are bound to deviate from it, but that such deviation is itself to be regarded as normal.)

2. Some idea of what a woman might expect to feel at varying stages of labour, what her response might be, how she might cope, and how her companion might help. (Information of this sort, provided that it is accurate, has been shown to be highly effective in helping an individual cope with a stressful event.[3])

   Part of this might include relaxation techniques in a variety of positions, so that the woman learns to release tension from the muscles she is not using. Different muscles will be used according to the posture the woman adopts, and part of enabling a woman to select her own positions freely in labour is ensuring that she practices relaxation and breathing techniques in a variety of positions, e.g. standing, kneeling, squatting, using a companion for support etc. If women are not encouraged to try out different positions in practice, they are less likely to try them in labour.

3. Breathing techniques. These are not magical devices for ensuring pain-free labour, and should not be offered as such. Early teaching, based on psychoprophylaxis, which aimed to teach a woman how to control her labour, and which could induce profound feelings of failure if she subsequently experienced pain in labour,[4] has now been largely superseded in Britain by a more physiological approach to the teaching of breathing in labour. Observations of labouring mammals (including human females) reveal that breathing is unremarkable in the early stages of labour, but usually becomes progressively faster and shallower as labour progresses, (often accompanied by restless behaviour), culminating in rapid breathing punctuated by short episodes of grunting and/or breath-holding. The physiological response to pain or fear is often prolonged breath-holding or gasping, neither of which, if continued over any length of time, is of benefit to either the woman or her baby. Thus an awareness of the sort of

pattern a woman might expect her breathing to develop as labour progresses, coupled with discussion of what she might be feeling and what might be happening within her, may be helpful to her in a society where she has not had the opportunity of becoming familiar with women's responses to labour as she grew up. There are various ways of approaching the teaching of this 'awareness' (using images of levels, spirals, waves etc.), all of which are means to this end. There are those who feel that any sort of instruction in breathing for labour is unnecessary and even counter-productive,[5] and this may be true if a woman is able to deliver in a calm, supportive, sensitive environment in which her individual needs take priority. In such a place it is likely that each labouring woman will be entirely free to discover her body's own coping mechanisms and labour 'intuitively'. However such optimal environments are rarely found in British hospitals.

4. As should be clear from previous chapters, a woman's perception of labour does not hinge on the presence or absence of pain, and even the 'best' labours are stressful.

> . . . So the whole labour lasted 5 hours, but the 'cost' of such a brief labour was its fierceness. The contractions built up so quickly and I was really knocked sideways by the intensity of the physical sensations, but it wasn't pain (except during the birth of her head). I almost doubted my ability to carry on at times . . .

Thus classes often include a consideration of some of the other ways a woman may be helped to cope. Effleurage (a form of light stroking), massage, and the use of heat and/or cold as counter-irritants are all consistent with the gate theory of pain, which proposes that pain impulses can be blocked by stimuli from other nerve pathways not involved in pain transmission.[6] It is possible that transcutaneous electrical nerve stimulation (TENS) works on this principle. It is also possible that part of its effect is due to its enhancement of endorphin release in the brain. Schachter[6] reports that several studies have shown that acupuncture increases the levels of endorphins in the spinal fluid, and this too can provide effective non-invasive, non-pharmacological analgesia.

5. Some classes, particularly in areas where women find it difficult to negotiate the sort of birth they want, may include some assertiveness training and role-play.

Perhaps the success or otherwise of a course of classes should not be measured by the details of the obstetric outcomes of the woman who participated, but by the extent to which each woman felt prepared for labour beforehand, and the extent to which the actual experience conformed to her expectations and her image of herself. Within a single group there may be women with both very low expectations, who are fearful and pessimistic, and those with very high expectations who think that 'positive attitudes in pregnancy bring about a painless, peak-experience kind of labour and who have high ego involvement in labour going a certain pre-determined way'.[7] The antenatal teacher has the difficult task of raising the confidence of the first group and enabling them to discover personal resources of which they were unaware, in order to avoid their approach to labour leading them realize their worst fears; while in the same setting bringing the expectations of the second group to focus within a more realistic framework.

It is the complexity of these factors that has led two researchers[7] to suggest that the more childbirth education classes can be tailored to take account of individual differences, the better, with each woman attending known as an individual to the person taking the classes.

This can rarely be achieved within the NHS at present, but is quite compatible with the concept of 'continuity of care' team midwifery schemes, if antenatal education is seen as an important part of antenatal care.

Birth Plans

Some women, particularly those who have read widely and carefully planned their pregnancy, have a fairly clear idea of what they expect from their care-givers from very early on; for others their possible options and their reactions to them become apparent gradually as their pregnancy progresses. Unless the woman is content to leave all the decision-making to her attendants, she will at some point have to communicate her hopes and concerns to them. Midwives and obstetricians are not mind readers; if the woman does not say what she wants, the best they can do is to give her the sort of care that they genuinely believe to be in her best interests. (Assuming of course that they do not initiate the discussion themselves!) At worst the woman will be subjected to the routines of the institution/obstetrician/ midwife regardless of her individual requirements.

Most women, especially those pregnant for the first time, will have some anxieties and questions. One of the ways in which they can ensure that when faced with their care-givers (possibly after a long wait in a busy clinic) they do not forget what they were going to say, is to write it down. If a woman does have strong feelings about any aspect of her care, particularly during the labour itself, it should be discussed beforehand—labour is no time to be arguing with the obstetrician or midwife. If the woman's attendants during labour will not be those who have seen her antenatally, any relevant instructions/requests can be recorded in the notes, or wherever those caring for her will see them. A 'memory aid' of this sort is rather different from what is commonly understood as a 'birth plan'.

A birth plan is a more formal, written statement of what the woman or couple wish to have happen in labour and in the days following it. One copy is put into the notes and the woman keeps a copy herself. Ideally, the creation of a birth plan should be part of a process, enabling a woman to come to terms with the approach of birth and parenthood, and encouraging her to increase her understanding and knowledge of what is involved. In this respect it can be seen as a means of enhancing her growing sense of responsibility for herself and her child. Unfortunately it is much more commonly used by women as an attempt to gain a greater sense of control in a situation in which they feel they have very little; an attempt to focus the attention of care-givers on an individual woman in a situation in which she feels she is just another name.

Maternity care professionals, by definition, deal with parturient women every day, and it may be hard for them to ensure that their care always reflects the uniqueness of each woman's birth. If they also work in an institution it is even easier for them to allow administrative concerns to take priority. (Those who see women in a more social context are often less constrained.)

At its most basic level a birth plan may consist of a series of written instructions to caregivers to abstain from intervention, e.g. 'I do not want and do not consent to the following . . .' and it is an indictment of the system of care and the individuals that perpetuate it if there is so little willingness/opportunity/time for women to discuss their anxieties that they feel that they have to resort to such undiplomatic statements. Unfortunately this approach is also the one most likely to be resented by obstetricians and midwives, partly because it assumes that unless restrained they would realize the woman's worst fears, and partly because, in some forms, such a birth plan may tie their hands if labour deviates from normal, or if the baby needs special care. Should emergencies arise, whether at home or in hospital, the woman should give her care-givers the same co-operation that she would expect from them in a straightforward birth.

Not all professionals, however, regard birth plans as threatening. In hospitals where the rigid protocol of the labour ward creates conflict within midwives as they try to balance the obligations of their Code of Practice with the needs of an individual woman, birth plans can help to reduce the pressure on the midwife by providing a legitimate means of ignoring the protocol.[8]

Some hospitals may try to pre-empt birth plans by producing their own. At worst these re-assert the power of the institution by defining and limiting the choices that are available. In this situation the woman may be given a menu-style plan with a list of options from which to choose. Often these ignore or trivialize the fundamental issues of responsibility and control ('do you want to wear your own nightgown in labour?') or leave no room for discussion or manoeuvre ('do you wish to have analgesia?')

At best they can be incorporated into a guide to labour; setting out in reasonable detail the way things are normally done at the hospital. If this is coupled, at a later date, with time set aside to discuss this and to enable each woman to make specific additions, omissions or alterations, it has the dual advantage of reducing both maternal and professional anxiety.

Some consumer organizations produce sample birth plans for women to use as a guide when constructing their own, with suggestions of the sort of questions they might want to ask.[9] These may be useful in conjunction with locally or nationally compiled information, based on hospital statistics and/or womens' experiences about the flexibility and policies of various institutions and systems of care.[10] Such plans should be couched in general (but not vague) terms, reflecting the positive aspects of the woman's preferences ('I hope to be able to . . .' rather than 'I do not want . . .') and allowing for the possibility that the woman may change her mind in labour.

It is unreasonable to ask for or expect any prior commitment to any pattern of labour from a woman, as no one can know how she will respond to her labour. The terms 'active birth' or 'natural birth' are appropriately used, in at least one hospital[11] to describe birth retrospectively; an active birth being one in which alternative birth positions were used, but which does not preclude the use of drugs, and a natural birth being one in which no drugs were used but which may or may not have been active. Retrospective categorization may have its critics, but it does not limit or constrain a woman in the process of giving birth. No doubt many women seeking the kind of birth advocated by Odent[12] would welcome the knowledge that they would not be offered 'artificial' ways of coping with labour (pethidine, epidurals etc.), but that is not the same as providing an environment in which they may not ask for them, should they feel the need; with the proviso that they fully understand their limitations and side-effects.

Paradoxically, units where the approach to labour care is flexible and sensitive, or where there is both the time and the inclination to listen to and discuss women's feelings with regard to the conduct of their labour, are also the units where birth plans as 'intervention insurance' are least likely to be needed.

If women feel that the only way they have of protecting themselves in units with fixed protocols for normal labour is to produce a birth plan relating to aspects of care that have been neither discussed nor negotiated antenatally, then the birth plan is being used as a substitute for trust. Klein has noted that women who do this often end up with more, rather than fewer, of the interventions that they sought to avoid.[13] This may be because women who cannot trust their attendants in labour cannot let go emotionally, allowing their minds and bodies to focus exclusively on the process of labour, in the manner described in earlier chapters. Women in this situation might fare better if their time and emotional energy were put into finding alternative givers or systems of care in which the relationship could be based on trust rather than on fear.

There is very little need for a birth plan in situations where women receive all their pregnancy, labour and postnatal care from the same midwife or small group of midwives, except perhaps at the level of a convenient set of reminders. Thus birth plans are perhaps most useful in the antenatal period, where they can serve to identify the basic philosophies and flexibility of the care-givers, and to reveal any important areas of disagreement, at a time when it is still possible to find alternative care.

In the context of a caring relationship, usually between women and midwives, the development of a birth plan might be used as a positive learning experience. Used in this way it could be added to and modified as the pregnancy progressed, reflecting the woman's growing self-confidence and awareness of the reality of birth. This sort of plan would not be a prescription for labour, but would be evidence not only of the woman's preferences, but also of her contingency plans, should labour require that she take a different course of action from the one she had anticipated.

Giving birth is not a process that can be detached from other aspects of a woman's life; it is part of a continuum; intimately bound up with how she feels about her body, her relationship with others, her role as a woman, her sense of identity. This is true for all births, straightforward or otherwise, and one of the reasons why the circumstances of birth are so important, and safety and satisfaction are indissolubly linked. Neither is it a matter of success or failure, but of realizing the full potential of each individual. There is no insurmountable reason why every woman should not be able to have the sort of birth that she can look back on as the best she could achieve. For some women this will not preclude regrets, but for all it could be a positive, enriching experience.

Appendix 1 Risk Factors

The indications for hospital confinement have grown considerably in the last fifteen years, and in Holland, which still has the highest home-confinement rate in the developed world, as well as one of the lowest perinatal mortality rates, the absence of all of the following indications is now officially a precondition for home confinement, as it is in most of the UK.

However, in reality, these 'indicators of risk'[1] are more usefully regarded as guidelines, and decisions need to be made on an individual basis taking the whole of the woman's circumstances into account, not simply on the presence or absence of a 'risk factor'. Many of these factors are readily negotiable: age for example, depending on the circumstances and/or the motivation of the woman.

1. A woman expecting her first child (a primigravida), who is over 30 years of age.

2. A woman expecting her second or subsequent child (a multigravida), who is over 35 years of age.

3. A woman expecting her fourth or subsequent child. This is held to be a risk factor, although unpublished observations from the 1958 British Perinatal Mortality Survey show that, providing that the preceding pregnancies have been uneventful, this group are not 'at risk' if they are not over 35 years of age.

4. Low social class. In Britain; a woman who falls into social class IV or V as defined by the Office of Population Censuses and Surveys. This is a very broad classification and has to be interpreted in the light of the individual woman's environment.

5. Disorders of maternal growth; in particular women who are (a) small or (b) grossly overweight.

   (a) A height of less than 158 cms (5 ft 2 ins) is associated with a higher perinatal mortality rate. This is probably because women in lower income groups are more likely to fail to reach the full height of which they are potentially capable, by virtue of a poor environment or an unsatisfactory diet. The fact that the majority of perinatal deaths to women in this category are not due solely to mechanical causes (i.e. disproportion, or the woman's pelvis being too small to allow the baby's head to pass through) supports this explanation.

   (b) Definitions of obesity vary, but a commonly used criterion is a weight of between 175 – 250 lbs, depending on the outcome measure being studied. Obese women are considerably more at risk of developing complications in pregnancy and thus moving into category 13 below. Hypertension, gestational diabetes, and pre-eclampsia are all significantly more likely to arise in obese women. Some studies suggest that the incidence of operative delivery, wound and urinary infections, thromboembolism, deep vein thrombosis and malpresentation is likely to be increased in such women.[2-9]

6. A woman who has rhesus problems or other forms of isoimmunization. (This does not mean all women who are rhesus negative, only those who have circulating antibodies).

7. A woman who has had an operation on her uterus, e.g. a previous caesarean section, removal of fibroids (myomectomy) or a previous hysterotomy to terminate a pregnancy. This again does not mean that a woman in this category cannot have a perfectly normal delivery,[10] but simply that

the scar on her uterus will need careful 'watching' during labour—if it gave way, an immediate caesarean section would be necessary.

8. Previous third stage problems. A history of a retained placenta or a postpartum haemorrhage (bleeding after the birth of a baby resulting in a blood loss of 1–1½ or more pints) are usually regarded as strong indications for hospital delivery, as there is evidence that these problems are more likely to occur in a woman who has once had such problems, even if intervening third stages have been normal.[11] However there is also a suggestion that some third stage problems are iatrogenic, and there is (again) scope for making decisions on an individual basis.[12,13]

9. A woman with a bad obstetric history, e.g. previous forceps deliveries, premature labours, etc,

10. Previous low birth weight babies: this includes not only babies born prematurely, but also those who failed to grow properly in the uterus ('small for dates' or 'dysmature'). Babies in this group account for over 50 per cent of all perinatal deaths.

11. Coexisting maternal illness, e.g. high blood pressure, renal disease, diabetes.

12. Any woman who has received no antenatal care. Women in this category are automatically considered to be 'at risk', as none of the potential risk elements will have been ruled out.

13. Any condition which may develop during the course of the pregnancy which may move the mother into a higher risk category:

    (a) Pre-eclampsia (sometimes called toxaemia of pregnacy). This is normally considered to be present when two out of the three usually associated symptoms are present— a rise in diastolic blood pressure of more than 20 mmHg pressure above the 'booking' blood pressure, or a rise above 100 mmHg; protein in the urine (proteinuria); and fluid retention (oedema).

(b) Antepartum haemorrhage (bleeding from the placental site).

(c) Malpresentation. Any position of the baby other then head first, e.g. breech, shoulder or transverse lie; or head first but with the face or forehead (brow) lying over the cervix (instead of the back or top of the head).

(d) Fetal growth retardation. 'Diagnosed' usually because the uterus is not expanding at the expected rate, or the baby seems smaller then expected for the stage of pregnancy. This finding usually promps further investigation. (However there is some evidence that this condition is over-diagnosed; in one study[14] there were 2.5 false positives for every case correctly diagnosed (see page 59).

(e) Poor maternal weight gain. A weight gain of less than 9 kg (20 lbs) may prompt further investigation as the 1972 US Collaborative study has indicated that a weight gain of 9 – 14 kgs (20 – 35 lb) is the range within which there is the lowest rate of perinatal mortality and delivery of low birth weight babies.[15]

It follows from the above that a woman who is over 5 ft 2 in, under 30 years of age having her first baby; or a woman who is over 5 ft 2 in, under 35 years of age and having her second or subsequent baby, in social class I, II or III, and with no medical or obstetric problems is in a category of 'low risk' and could if she so desired have her baby at home or in a GP unit which is not part of a consultant maternity hospital. (As stated before, the fact that she does not meet these criteria in all respects does not mean that she is automatically ineligible. Ultimately, each woman can decide for herself where she will have her baby).

Appendix 2 Community Midwifery Services for England and Wales

The National Health Service is now administered through fifteen main Regional Health Authorities in England and Wales. Each Region is further sub-divided into Districts, and in each district there is a 'base' from which a community midwifery service of some sort will operate. The exact nature of the service will vary from district to district.

Listed below is the address and phone number for each base in each District Health Authority, for each Region. Ask for, or write to, the Senior Midwife, Community Midwifery Services.

East Anglian Regional Health Authority

Cambridge DHA (District Health Authority)   Rosie Maternity Hospital, Robinson Way, Cambridge CB2 2SW. Tel. 0223 245151.
East Suffolk DHA   Ipswich Hospital, Heath Road Wing, Ipswich IP4 5PD. Tel. 0473 712233.
Great Yarmouth and Waveney DHA   James Paget Hospital, Lowestoft Road, Gorleston, Great Yarmouth NR31 6LA Tel. 0493 600611.
Huntingdon DHA   Hinchinbrooke Hospital, Hinchinbrooke Park, Huntingdon, Cambridgeshire PE18 8NT. Tel. 0480 56131.
Norwich DHA   St. Michael's Hospital, Aylsham, Norwich NR11 6NA. Tel. 0263 732341.
Peterborough DHA   Maternity Unit, Alderman's Drive, Peterborough PE3 6BP. Tel. 0733 67451.
West Norfolk and Wisbech DHA   Queen Elizabeth Hospital, Gayton Road, Kings Lynn PE30 4ET. Tel. 0553 766266.

West Suffolk DHA   West Suffolk Hospital, Hardwick Lane, Bury St Edmonds IP33 2QZ. Tel. 0284 63131.

Mersey Regional Health Authority

Chester DHA   Maternity Unit, Countess of Chester Hospital, Liverpool Road, Chester CH1 2BA. Tel. 0244 315500.

Crewe DHA   Leighton Hospital, Middlewich Road, Crewe CW1 4QJ. Tel. 0270 255141.

Halton DHA   Victoria House, The Holloway, Runcorn WA7 4TH. Tel. 0928 714567.

Liverpool DHA   Nurses Home, Mill Road Maternity Hospital, Liverpool L6 2AH. Tel. 051 260 8787.

Macclesfield DHA   West Park Hospital, Prestbury Road, Macclesfield, SK10 3BL. Tel. 0625 21000.

St. Helen's and Knowsley DHA   Maternity Unit, Whiston Hospital, Prescot, L35 5DR. Tel. 051 426 1600.

Southport and Formby DHA   Christina Hartley Maternity Hospital, Curzon Road, Southport PR8 6PL. Tel. 0704 42901.

South Sefton (Merseyside) DHA   Maternity Unit, Fazakerley Hospital, Longmoor Lane, Liverpool L9 7AL. Tel. 051 525 5980.

Warrington DHA   Maternity Unit, Warrington District General Hospital, Lovely Lane, Warrington WA5 1QG. Tel. 0925 35911.

Wirral DHA   St Catherine's Hospital, Church Road, Birkenhead L42 0LQ. Tel. 051 678 5111.

Northern Regional Health Authority

Darlington DHA   Greenbank Maternity Hospital, Greenbank Road, Darlington DL3 6EW. Tel. 0325 380100.

Durham DHA   Midwifery Dept, Dryburn Hospital, North Road, Durham DH1 5TW. Tel. 091 386 4911.

East Cumbria DHA   City Maternity Hospital, Fusehill Street, Carlisle, Cumbria. Tel. 0228 23444.

Gateshead DHA   Maternity Unit, Queen Elizabeth's Hospital, Gateshead NE9 6SX. Tel. 091 487 8989.

Hartlepool DHA   Cameron Hospital, Wooler Road, Hartlepool. Tel. 0429 266654.

Newcastle DHA   Princess Mary's Maternity Hospital, Great North Road, Newcastle-upon-Tyne NE2 3BD. Tel. 091 281 4506.

North Tees DHA   Maternity Unit, North Tees General Hospital, Hardwick, Stockton-on-Tees TS19 8PE. Tel. 0642 672122.

North Tyneside DHA North Tyneside General Hospital, Rake Lane, North Shields NE29 8NH. Tel. 091 259 6660.

Northumberland DHA Ashington Hospital, West View, Ashington NE63 0SA. Tel. 0670 812541.

North-West Durham DHA Maternity Dept, Shotley Bridge General Hospital, Consett, County Durham, DH8 0NB. Tel. 0207 503456.

South Cumbria DHA
(1) Furness: Maternity Unit, Furness General Hospital, Dalton Lane, Barrow-in-Furness LA14 4LF. Tel. 0229 32020.
(2) South Lakeland: Helme Chase Maternity Hospital, Kendal. Tel. 0539 21406.

South Tees DHA Middlesborough Maternity Hospital, Park Road North, Middlesborough TS1 3LE. Tel. 0642 245156.

South Tyneside DHA Maternity Unit, General Hospital, Harton Lane, South Shields NE34 0PL. Tel. 091 456 1161.

South West Durham DHA Midwifery Unit, Bishop Auckland General Hospital, Bishop Auckland, County Durham DL14 6AD. Tel. 0388 604040.

Sunderland DHA
(1) North: Hylton Castle Health Centre, Coleridge Road, Sunderland SR5 3PP. Tel. 091 549 5016.
(2) South-east: Monkswearmouth Health Centre, Dundas Street, Sunderland SR6 0BD. Tel. 091 514 0431.
(3) South-west: Alderman Jack Cohen Health Centre, Springwell Road, Sunderland SR3 4DX. Tel. 091 528 2828.

West Cumbria DHA Maternity Unit, West Cumberland Hospital, Hensingham, Whitehaven CA28 8JG. Tel. 0946 3181.

North-Western Regional Health Authority

Blackburn Hyndburn and Ribble Valley DHA Queen's Park Hospital, Haslingden Road, Blackburn BB2 3HH. Tel. 0254 63555.

Blackpool, Wyre and Fylde DHA Maternity Unit, Victoria Hospital, Whinney Heys Road, Blackpool FY3 8NR. Tel. 0253 34111.

Bolton DHA Princess Anne Maternity Unit, Bolton General Hospital, Minerva Road, Farnworth, Bolton. Tel. 0204 390573.

Burnley, Pendle and Rossendale DHA Edith Watson Maternity Unit, Burnley General Hospital, Casterton Avenue, Burnley BB10 2PQ. Tel. 0282 25071.

Bury DHA   Fairfield General Hospital, Jericho, Bury, Lancashire.
Tel. 061 7053706/7646081.

Central Manchester DHA   Radio-Telephone Room, St Mary's
Hospital, Manchester M13 0JH. Tel. 061 2761234.

Chorley and South Ribble DHA   Maternity Unit, Chorley and
District Hospital, Preston Road, Chorley, Lancashire PR7 1PP.
Tel. 0257 265555.

Lancaster DHA   Maternity Unit, Royal Lancaster Infirmary,
Ashton Road, Lancaster LA1 4RP. Tel. 0524 65944.

North Manchester DHA   Midwifery Unit, North Manchester
General Hospital, Crumpsall, Manchester M8 6RL.
Tel. 061 795 4567.

Oldham DHA   Ground Floor, Marron Maternity Unit, Oldham
District General Hospital, Rochdale Road, Oldham OL1 2JH.
Tel. 061 652 5811.

Preston DHA   Sharoe General Hospital, Fulwood, Preston PR2
4DU. Tel. 0772 716525.

Rochdale DHA   Birch Hill Hospital, Rochdale OL12 9QB.
Tel. 0706 77777.

Salford DHA   Midwifery Unit, Hope Hospital, Salford M6 8HD.
Tel. 061 789 7373.

South Manchester DHA
North: Withington Maternity Unit, Nell Lane, Manchester M20
8LR. Tel. 061 447 4223/4233.
South: Wythenshawe Maternity Unit, Southmoor Road,
Manchester M23 9LT. Tel. 061 998 7070.

Stockport DHA   Maternity Unit, Stepping Hill Hospital, Poplar
Grove, Stockport SK2 7JE. Tel. 061 483 1010.

Tameside and Glossop DHA   Maternity Unit, Tameside General
Hospital, Fountain Street, Ashton-under-Lyne, Lancashire OL6
9RW. Tel. 061 330 8373.

Trafford DHA   Park Hospital, Davyhulme, Manchester M31 3SL.
Tel. 061 748 4022.

West Lancashire DHA   Midwifery Dept, Ormskirk and District
General Hospital, Wigan Road, Ormskirk, Lancashire L39 2AZ.
Tel. 0695 75471.

Wigan DHA   The Bungalow, Billinge Hospital, Up Holland Road,
Wigan, WN5 7ET. Tel. 0695 632855.

Oxfordshire Regional Health Authority

Aylesbury Vale DHA   Royal Buckinghamshire Hospital,
Aylesbury, HP19 3AB. Tel. 0296 84111.
East Berkshire DHA
South: Heatherwood Hospital, Ascot SL5 8AA. Tel. 0990 23333.
North: Ward 22, Wexham Park Hospital, Slough SL2 4HL.
Tel. 0753 34567.
Kettering DHA
(1) Maternity Unit, Kettering General Hospital, Rothwell Road,
Kettering NN16 8UZ. Tel. 0536 81141.
(2) Midwives Office, Irthlingborough Road, Wellingborough,
Northamptonshire. Tel. 0933 225033.
(3) Midwives Office, Willowbrook Health Centre, Cottingham
Road, Corby, Northamptonshire. Tel. 0536 64211.
Milton Keynes DHA   Maternity Dept, Milton Keynes General
Hospital, Standing Way, Eaglestone, Milton Keynes MK6 5LD.
Tel. 0908 660033.
Northampton DHA   Barratt Maternity Home, General Hospital,
Northampton NN1 5BD. Tel. 0604 34700.
Oxfordshire DHA   Level 5, John Radcliffe Hospital (1),
Headington, Oxford OX3 9DU. Tel. 0865 64711.
West Berkshire DHA   Maternity Unit, Royal Berkshire Hospital,
Craven Road, Reading RG1 5AN. Tel. 0734 875111.
Wycombe DHA   Midwifery Unit, Wycombe General Hospital,
Queen Alexandra Road, High Wycombe HP11 2TT.
Tel. 0494 26161.

Special Regional Health Authority

Hammersmith and Queen Charlotte's Hospital Special
Queen Charlotte's Maternity Hospital, Goldhawk Road, London,
W6 0XG. Tel. 01 748 4666.

South-Western Regional Health Authority

Bristol and Weston DHA
(1) Bristol Maternity Hospital, Southwell Street, Bristol BS2 8EG.
Tel. 0272 215411.
(2) Maternity Unit, Weston General Hospital, Uphill, Weston-
super-Mare, Avon. Tel. 0934 636363.

Cheltenham and District DHA

(1) Cheltenham: St. Paul's Hospital, Swindon Road, Cheltenham GL50 4BW. Tel. 0242 516291.

(2) Tewkesbury: Community Nursing Offices, Health Centre, Newton Road, Cheltenham GL51 7QX. Tel. 0242 525800.

(3) Cotswold: Community Nursing Service, The Clinic, Watermoor Road, Cirencester, Gloucestershire GL7 1JS. Tel. 0285 69477.

Cornwall and Isles of Scilly DHA

(1) Community Unit HQ, Penrice Hospital, Porthpean Road, St Austell, Cornwall PL26 6AA. Tel 0726 68232.

(2) Health Office, Moorland Road, St. Austell, Cornwall. Tel. 0726 72206.

(3) Health Office, Camborne. Tel. 0209 714221.

Exeter DHA

(1) Exeter City: Royal Devon and Exeter Hospital, Heavitree, Exeter EX1 2ED. Tel. 0392 50541.

(2) Tiverton: Bungalow, Belmont Hospital, Tiverton. Tel. 0884 258123.

(3) Cullompton: Health Centre, Exeter Hill, Cullompton. Tel. 0884 33766.

(4) Honiton and area: Honiton Hospital, Honiton. Tel. 0404 2362.

(5) Ottery St Mary: Ottery St Mary Hospital. Tel. 0404 812188.

(6) Axminster and area: Axminster Hospital. Tel. 0297 32071.

(7) Seaton and Beer: Health Centre, Harepath Road, Seaton. Tel. 0297 20877.

(8) Sidmouth and area: Victoria Cottage Hospital, Sidmouth. Tel. 0395 52482.

(9) Exmouth and Budleigh Salterton: Exmouth Hospital, Exmouth. Tel. 0395 279684.

(10) Okehampton: Castle Hospital, Okehampton. Tel. 0837 2411.

Frenchay DHA   Chipping Sodbury Maternity Hospital, Bristol. Tel. 0454 323824.

Gloucester DHA

(1) Gloucester City: Maternity Unit, Gloucestershire Royal Hospital, Great Western Road, Gloucester G41 3NN. Tel. 0452 28555.

(2) Stroud: Stroud General Hospital, Stroud, Gloucestershire. Tel. 0453 62283.

(3) Forest of Dean: 24 Grove Road, Lydney, Gloucestershire. Tel. 0594 42518.

North Devon DHA   Maternity Unit, Devon District Hospital, Pilton, Barnstaple EX31 4JB. Tel. 0271 72577.

Plymouth DHA   Ward 11a, Freedom Fields Maternity Unit, Plymouth PL4 8QQ. Tel. 0752 834217/8.

Somerset DHA
(1) Taunton Town: GP Unit, Musgrove Park Hospital, Taunton. Tel. 0823 333444.
(2) Bridgewater: Mary Stanley Maternity Hospital, Bridgewater. Tel. 0278 422614.
(3) Chard: Chard and District Hospital, Chard TA20 1NF. Tel. 0460 63175.
(4) Minehead: Minehead Hospital, The Avenue, Minehead TA24 5LY. Tel. 0643 3377.
(5) Wells: Wells and District General Hospital, Wells, BA5 2XL. Tel. 0749 73154.
(6) Yeovil: Maternity Unit, Yeovil District Hospital, Higher Kingston, Yeovil BA21 4AT. Tel. 0935 75122.

Southmead DHA   A Block, Maternity Unit, Southmead Hospital, Westbury-on-Trym, Bristol BS10 5NB. Tel. 0272 505050.

Torbay DHA   Maternity Unit, Torbay Hospital, Lawes Bridge, Torquay TQ2 7AA. Tel. 0803 64567.

North-east Thames Regional Health Authority

Barking, Havering and Brentwood DHA
(1) Rush General Hospital, Dagenham Road, Romford RM7 0YA. Tel. 0708 46066.
(2) Harold Wood Hospital, Gubbins Lane, Harold Wood, Romford RM3 0BE. Tel. 04023 45533.

Basildon and Thurrock DHA   Basildon Hospital, Nethermayne, Basildon, SS16 5NL. Tel. 0268 3911.

Bloomsbury DHA   Obstetrics Hospital, University College Hospital, Huntley Street, London WC1E 6AU. Tel. 01 380 9567.

City and Hackney DHA   Hackney/Homerton Unit, Hackney Hospital, Homerton High Street, London E9. Tel. 01 985 6822/5555.

Enfield DHA   Maternity Dept, Chase Farm Hospital, The Ridgeway, Enfield, Middlesex EN2 8JL. Tel. 01 366 6600.

Hampstead DHA   Obstetric Unit, Royal Free Hospital, Pond Street, London, NW3 2QG. Tel. 01 794 0500.

Haringey DHA   North Middlesex Hospital, Midwifery Unit, Sterling Way, Edmonton, London N18 1QX.
Tel. 01 807 7097/ 71.

Islington DHA   City of London Maternity Unit, Whittington
Hospital, Highgate Hill, London N19 5NF. Tel. 01 272 3070/5196.
Mid Essex DHA   St John's Hospital, Chelmsford CM2 9BG.
Tel. 0245 25 2666.
Newham DHA   Maternity Unit, Newham General Hospital, Glen
Road, Plaistow, London, E13 8SL. Tel. 01 476 1400.
North East Essex DHA
(1) Colchester, Halstead, Tiptree, Wivenhoe: Colchester Maternity
Hospital, 32–4 Lexden Road, Colchester. Tel. 0206 65864.
(2) Coastal, Clacton, Harwich: Clacton and District Hospital,
Clacton-on-Sea. Tel. 0255 421145/421235.
Redbridge DHA   King George's Hospital, West Wing, Eastern
Avenue, Newbury Park, Ilford, IG2 7RL. Tel. 01 518 2299.
Southend DHA   Maternity Unit, Rochford Hospital, Dalys Road,
Rochford SS4 1RB. Tel. 0702 546393.
Tower Hamlets DHA   The London Hospital (Mile End), 275
Bancroft Road, London E1 4DG. Tel. 01 558 0234.
Waltham Forest DHA   Maternity Unit, Whipps Cross Hospital,
Leytonstone, London E11 1NR. Tel. 01 539 5522.
West Essex DHA   Princess Alexandra Hospital, Hamstel Road,
Harlow CM20 1QX. Tel. 0279 26791.

North-west Thames Regional Health Authority

Barnet DHA   Community Office, C Wing, Victoria Maternity
Hospital, Wood Street, Barnet, EN5 4BG. Tel. 01 441 2050/5111.
Brent DHA   Maternity Unit, Central Middlesex Hospital, Acton
Lane, London NW10 7NS. Tel. 01 965 5733.
Ealing DHA   Perivale Maternity Hospital, Stockdove Way,
Greenford, Middlesex UB6 8EL. Tel 01 997 5661.
East Hertfordshire DHA   Dept of Midwifery, Queen Elizabeth II
Hospital, Welwyn Garden City AL7 4HQ. Tel 0707 328111.
Harrow DHA   Northwick Park Hospital, Watford Road, Harrow
HA1 3UJ. Tel 01 864 5311.
Hillingdon DHA   Hillingdon Hospital, Uxbridge UB8 3NN.
Tel. 0895 38282.
Hounslow and Spelthorne DHA   92 Bath Road, Hounslow TW3
3EL. Tel. 01 570 7715.
North Bedfordshire DHA   North Wing, Bedford General
Hospital, 3 Kimbolton Road, Bedford MK40 2NU.
Tel. 0234 55122.

North Hertfordshire DHA   Maternity Unit, Lister Hospital, Coreys Mill Lane, Stevenage SG1 4RT. Tel. 0438 314333.

North West Hertfordshire DHA

(1) Harpenden, London Colney, Markyate, Redbourn, St. Albans: St Alban's City Hospital, Maternity Unit, Normandy Road, St Alban's, Hertfordshire. Tel. 0727 66122.

(2) Berkhamstead, Bovingdon, Chipperfield, Hemel Hempstead, Kings Langley, Tring: Hemel Hempstead General Hospital, St Paul's Wing, Maternity Unit, Allandale, Hemel Hempstead. HP2 5HT. Tel. 0442 3141.

Paddington and North Kensington DHA   St Mary's Hospital, Praed Street, London W2 1NY. Tel. 01 725 6666/1131.

Riverside DHA

(1) Hammersmith and Fulham: Queen Charlotte's Maternity Hospital, Goldhawk Road, London W6 0XG. Tel. 01 748 4666.

(2) Victoria: Maternity Unit, Fifth Floor, Westminster Hospital, Dean Ryle Street, London SW1P 2AP.

South Bedfordshire DHA   Maternity Wing, Luton and Dunstable Hospital, Luton LU4 0DY. Tel. 0582 502002/491122.

South West Hertfordshire DHA   Maternity Wing, Watford General Hospital, Vicarage Road, Watford WD1 8HB. Tel. 0923 44366.

South-east Thames Regional Health Authority

Bexley DHA   Maternity Dept, Queen Mary's Hospital, Frognal Avenue, Sidcup DA14 6LT. Tel. 01 309 0391/302 2678.

Brighton DHA   Level 11, Tower Block, Royal Sussex County Hospital, Brighton BN2 5BE. Tel. 0273 969955.

Bromley DHA   Farnborough Hospital, Farnborough Common, Orpington BR6 8ND. Tel. 0689 62914/53333.

Camberwell DHA   Room 801, New Ward Block, Kings College Hospital, Denmark Hill, London SE5 9RS. Tel. 01 274 6222.

Canterbury and Thanet DHA   Maternity Dept, Kent and Canterbury Hospital, Ethelbert Road, Canterbury CT1 3NG. Tel. 0227 66877.

Dartford and Gravesham DHA

(1) Dartford: Dartford West Health Centre, Tower Road, Dartford DA1 2HA. Tel. 0322 73921.

(2) Gravesend: Community Nursing Office, Whitehall Clinic, Whitehall Road, Gravesend DA12 5HS. Tel. 0474 60099.

Eastbourne DHA District General Hospital, Kings Drive, Eastbourne BN21 2UD. Tel. 0323 21351/22744.

Greenwich DHA Devonport House, King William Walk, Greenwich, London SE10 9JH. Tel. 01 858 8090/8141.

Hastings DHA Buchanan Hospital, Springfield Road, St Leonards-on-Sea, East Sussex. Tel. 0424 422666.

Lewisham and North Southwark DHA

(1) Downham, Forest Hill, Hither Green, Lewisham, Sydenham: Midwifery Dept, Lewisham Hospital, High Street, Lewisham, London SE13. Tel. 01 690 4311/5036.

(2) Bermondsey, Deptford, North Southwark: McNair Centre, Guy's Hospital, London SE1. Tel. 01 407 7600.

Maidstone DHA Maidstone Hospital, Hermitage Lane, Barming, Maidstone ME16 9QQ. Tel. 0622 29000.

Medway DHA Canada House, Barnsole Road, Gillingham, Kent ME7 4JL. Tel. 0634 827117.

South-east Kent DHA Buckland Hospital, Coombe Valley Road, Buckland, Dover CT17 0HD. Tel. 0304 201624.

Tunbridge Wells DHA GP Unit, Pembury Hospital, Tunbridge Wells TN2 4QJ. Tel. 089 282 3535.

South-west Thames Regional Health Authority

Chichester DHA Maternity Unit, St Richard's Hospital, Spitalfield Lane, Chichester PO19 4SE. Tel. 0243 788122.

Croydon DHA Antenatal Clinic, Mayday Hospital, Mayday Road, Thornton Heath, Croydon CR4 7YE. Tel. 01 684 6999.

East Surrey DHA Maternity Unit, Redhill Hospital, Pendleton Road, Redhill RH1 6LA. Tel. 0737 765030.

Kingston and Esher DHA Averill Lodge, Kingston Hospital, Wolverton Avenue, Kingston, Surrey KT2 7QB. Tel. 01 546 7711.

Merton and Sutton DHA Maternity Unit, M Block, St Helier Hospital, Wrythe, Carshalton, Surrey. Tel. 01 641 1324.

Mid-Downs DHA

(1) East: Cuckfield Hospital, Ardingly Road, Cuckfield RH17 5HQ. Tel. 0444 459122.

(2) West: Crawley Hospital, West Green Drive, Crawley RH11 7DH. Tel. 0293 27866.

Mid-Surrey DHA Maternity Dept, Epsom District Hospital, Dorking Road, Epsom, Surrey. Tel. 03727 26100.

North-west Surrey DHA   Maternity Unit, St Peter's District General Hospital, Guildford Road, Chertsey KT16 0PZ. Tel. 093287 2000.

Richmond, Twickenham and Roehampton DHA   Midwifery Dept, Queen Mary's Hospital, Roehampton Lane, London SW15 5PN. Tel. 01 788 1350/789 6611.

South West Surrey DHA   St. Luke's Hospital, Warren Road, Guildford GU1 3LN. Tel. 0483 571122.

Wandsworth DHA   Midwifery Unit, Lanesborough Wing, St George's Hospital, Blackshaw Road, London SW17 0QT. Tel. 01 672 1255.

West Surrey and North-east Hampshire DHA   Community Office, Postnatal Ward, Frimley Park Hospital, Portsmouth Road, Frimley, Surrey GU16 5UT. Tel. 0276 62121.

Worthing District DHA   Southlands Hospital, Upper Shoreham Road, Shoreham-by-Sea, West Sussex. Tel. 0273 455622.

Trent Regional Health Authority

Barnsley DHA   Midwifery Area, Barnsley District General Hospital, Gawber Road, Barnsley, South Yorkshire. Tel. 0226 286122.

Bassetlaw DHA   Worksop Health Centre, Newgate Street, Worksop S80 1HP. Tel. 0909 476481.

Central Nottinghamshire DHA
(1) Priority Care: Dukeries Centre, Kings Mill Hospital, Mansfield Road, Sutton-in-Ashfield, NG17 4JL. Tel. 0623 22515.
(2) Newark: Newark General Hospital, London Road, Newark. Tel. 0636 73841.

Doncaster DHA   Maternity Dept, Doncaster Royal Infirmary, Doncaster DN2 5LT. Tel. 0302 66666.

Leicestershire DHA
(1) General Hospital: Leicester General Hospital, Leicester LE5 4PW. Tel. 0533 730222.
(2) Royal Infirmary: Leicester Royal Infirmary, Leicester LE1 5WW. Tel. 0533 541414.

North Derbyshire DHA   Scarsdale Hospital, Newbold Road, Chesterfield S41 7PF. Tel. 0246 77271.

North Lincolnshire DHA   Maternity Wing, County Hospital, Lincoln LN2 5QY. Tel. 0522 29921.

Nottingham DHA   Referral Unit, Memorial House, Standard Hill, Nottingham NG1 6FX. Tel. 0602 415333.

Rotherham DHA Obstetric Unit, Level B, Rotherham District General Hospital, Moorgate Road, Oakwood, Rotherham S60 2UD. Tel. 0709 362222.

Sheffield DHA Jessop Hospital for Women, Leavygreave Road, Sheffield S3 7RE. Tel. 0742 766333.

Southern Derbyshire DHA Ilkeston Maternity Home, Park Avenue, Ilkeston, Derbyshire DE7 5DM. Tel. 0602 301767.

South Lincolnshire DHA Pilgrim Hospital, Sibsey Road, Boston PE21 9QS. Tel. 0205 64801.

Wales Regional Health Authority

Clwyd DHA
(1) North: HM Stanley Hospital, St Asaph LL17 0RS.
Tel. 0745 593275.
(2) South: Maternity Unit, Maelor General Hospital, Wrexham LL13 7TD. Tel. 0978 353153.

East Dyfed DHA
(1) Carmarthen/Dinefwr: Community Health Services, West Wales General Hospital, Glangwilli, Carmarthen SA31 2AF.
Tel. 0267 235151.
(2) Ceredigion: Maternity Unit, Bronglais General Hospital, Aberystwyth. Tel. 0970 3131.
(3) Llanelli: Community Offices, Bryntirion Hospital, Swansea Road, Llanelli, SA15 3DX. Tel. 0554 774961.

Gwent DHA
(1) North: Nevill Hall Hospital, Abergavenny NP7 7EG.
Tel. 0873 2091.
(2) South: Room A10, Midwifery Dept, Royal Gwent Hospital, Newport NP9 2UB. Tel. 0633 52244.

Gwynedd DHA St David's Hospital, Bangor. Tel. 0248 370036.

Mid-Glamorgan DHA
(1) Merthyr/Cynon Valley: Merthyr General Hospital, Merthyr Tydfil. Tel. 0685 3651.
(2) Ogwr: Princess of Wales Hospital, Coity Road, Bridgend CF31 1RQ. Tel. 0656 62166.
(3) Rhondda: Community Health Office, Tyntyla Hospital, Ystrad, Rhondda CF41 7SS. Tel. 0443 436723.
(4) Rhymney Valley: Caerphilly District Miners' Hospital, St. Martin's Road, Caerphilly, CF8 2WW. Tel. 0222 851811.
(5) Taff Ely: East Glamorgan Hospital, Church Village, Pontypridd, CF38 1AB. Tel. 0443 204242.

Pembrokeshire DHA   Community Health Dept, Merlin's Hill, Haverfordwest, Pembrokeshire SA61 1PG. Tel. 0437 67801.

Powys DHA   Brecon War Memorial Hospital, Brecon, Powys. Tel. 0874 2443.

South Glamorgan DHA   St David's Hospital, Cowbridge Road East, Canton, Cardiff CF1 9TZ. Tel. 0222 44141.

West Glamorgan DHA   Central Clinic, 21 Orchard Street, Swansea. Tel. 0892 582054.

Wessex Regional Health Authority

Basingstoke and North Hampshire DHA   Shrubbery Floor, Maternity Dept, Basingstoke District Hospital, Aldermaston Road, Basingstoke RG24 9NA. Tel. 0256 465650.

Bath DHA
(1) Bath City/Bath Mansdyke: Princess Anne Wing, Royal United Hospital, Combe Park, Bath, Avon, BA1 3NG. Tel. 0225 28331.
(2) Frome: Frome Health Centre, Park Street, Frome, Somerset. Tel. 0373 62894.
(3) West and North West Wiltshire: The Health Clinic, The Halve, Trowbridge, Wiltshire. Tel. 022 146 6161.

East Dorset DHA   Poole General Hospital Maternity Unit, Longfleet Road, Poole BH15 2JB. Tel. 0202 675100.

Isle of Wight DHA   Obstetric Dept, St Mary's Hospital, Newport, Isle of Wight. Tel. 0983 524081.

Portsmouth and South-east Hampshire DHA   St Mary's Maternity Hospital, Milton, Portsmouth PO3 6AD. Tel. 0705 822331.

Salisbury DHA   Midwifery Unit, Odstock Hospital, Salisbury. Tel. 0722 336262.

Southampton and South-west Hampshire DHA   Princess Anne Hospital, Coxford Road, Southampton SO9 4HA. Tel. 0703 777222.

Swindon DHA   Maternity Unit, Princess Margaret Hospital, Okus Road, Swindon SN1 4JU. Tel. 0793 36231.

West Dorset DHA   West Dorset Hospital, Damers Road, Dorchester DT1 2JR. Tel. 0305 251150.

Winchester DHA   Florence Portal House, Royal Hampshire County Hospital, Winchester SO22 5DG. Tel. 0962 63535.

West Midlands Regional Health Authority

Bromsgrove and Redditch DHA   Bromsgrove and Redditch District General Hospital, Woodrow Drive, Redditch B98 7UB. Tel. 0527 503030.

Central Birmingham DHA   Birmingham Maternity Hospital, Queen Elizabeth Medical Centre, Birmingham B15 2TH. Tel. 021 472 1377.

Coventry DHA   Coventry Maternity Hospital, Clifford Bridge Road, Walsgrave, Coventry CV2 2DX. Tel. 0203 613232.

Dudley DHA   Midwifery Dept, Wordsley Hospital, Stourbridge, West Midlands DY8 5QX. Tel. 0384 288778.

East Birmingham DHA   Community Nursing Offices, East Birmingham Hospital, Yardley Green Unit, Yardley Green Road, Birmingham B9 5PX. Tel. 021 773 6422.

Herefordshire DHA   GP Unit, County Hospital, Hereford HR1 2ER. Tel. 0432 268161.

Kidderminster and District DHA   B Block, Kidderminster General Hospital, Bewdley Road, Kidderminster DY11 6RJ. Tel. 0562 3424.

Mid-Staffordshire DHA   Stafford District General Hospital, Westom Road, Stafford ST16 3SA. Tel. 0785 57731.

North Birmingham DHA   Community Health Office, Sutton Coldfield Hospital, 27a Birmingham Road, Sutton Coldfield B72 1QH. Tel. 021 354 2565.

North Staffordshire DHA   North Staffordshire Maternity Hospital, Hilton Road, Harpfields, Stoke-on-Trent ST4 6SD. Tel. 0782 621133.

North Warwickshire DHA   Nuneaton Maternity Hospital, Heath End Road, Nuneaton CV10 7DJ. Tel. 0203 384201.

Rugby DHA   Maternity Unit, Hospital of St Cross, Barby Road, Rugby CV22 5PX. Tel. 0788 72831.

Sandwell DHA   Sandwell District General Hospital, Lyndon, West Bromwich B71 4HJ. Tel. 021 553 1831.

Shropshire DHA   Royal Shrewsbury (Maternity) Hospital, Mytton Oak Road, Shrewsbury SY3 8XQ. Tel. 0743 231122.

Solihull DHA   Solihull Maternity Unit, Lode Lane, Solihull B91 2JL. Tel. 021 705 6741.

South Birmingham DHA   Sorrento Maternity Hospital, Wake Green Road, Moseley, Birmingham B13 3HE. Tel. 021 449 4242.

South-east Staffordshire DHA   Maternity Dept, Burton District Hospital Centre, Burton-on-Trent DE13 0RB. Tel. 0283 66333.

South Warwickshire DHA Cay Maternity Unit, Warneford Hospital, Radford Road, Leamington Spa CV31 1LU. Tel. 0926 27121.

Walsall DHA Manor Maternity Hospital, Moat Road, Walsall WS2 9PS. Tel. 0922 28911.

West Birmingham DHA Maternity Unit, Dudley Road Hospital, Birmingham B18 7QH. Tel. 021 551 6471/2.

Wolverhampton DHA Maternity Unit, New Cross Hospital, Wednesfield Road, Wolverhampton WV10 0QP. Tel. 0902 732255.

Worcester and District DHA Consultant Maternity Unit, Ronkswood Hospital, Newtown Road, Worcester WR5 1HN. Tel. 0905 763333.

Yorkshire Regional Health Authority

Airdale DHA Maternity Unit, Airdale General Hospital, Skipton Road, Steeton, Keighley, West Yorkshire BD20 6TD. Tel. 0535 52511.

Bradford DHA Maternity Unit, Bradford Royal Infirmary, Smith Lane, Bradford BD9 6RJ. Tel. 0274 42200.

Calderdale DHA Midwifery Unit, Halifax General Hospital, Halifax HX 0PW. Tel. 0422 57171.

Dewsbury DHA Staincliff Maternity Unit, Healds Road, Dewsbury WF13 4HS. Tel. 0924 465105.

East Yorkshire DHA East Riding General Hospital, Driffield, North Humberside YO25 7JR. Tel. 0377 42811.

Grimsby DHA Grimsby Maternity Hospital, Second Avenue, Nunsthorpe, Grimsby DN33 1NW. Tel. 0472 74111.

Harrogate DHA Maternity Unit, Harrogate General Hospital, Knaresborough Road, Harrogate HG2 7ND. Tel. 0423 885959.

Huddersfield DHA Antenatal Clinic, Huddersfield Royal Infirmary, Acre Street, Huddersfield HD3 3EA. Tel. 0484 20684/22191.

Hull DHA Maternity Hospital, Hedon Road, Hull HU9 5LX. Tel. 0482 76215.

Leeds Eastern DHA Clarendon Wing, Leeds General Infirmary, Blemond Grove, Leeds LS2 9NS. Tel. 0532 460388/432799.

Leeds Western DHA See Leeds Eastern.

Northallerton DHA Maternity Unit, Friargate Hospital, Northallerton DL6 1JG. Tel. 0609 779911.

Pontefract DHA   Maternity Unit, Pontefract General Infirmary, Friarwood Lane, Pontefract WF8 1PL. Tel. 0977 792361.

Scarborough DHA   Maternity Unit, Scarborough Hospital, Scalby Road, Scarborough YO12 6QL. Tel. 0723 368111.

Scunthorpe DHA   Maternity Home, Brumby Wood Lane, Scunthorpe, South Humberside DN17 1RF. Tel. 0724 282282.

Wakefield DHA   Manygates Hospital, Barnsley Road, Wakefield WF1 5NS. Tel. 0924 255021.

York DHA   Maternity Unit, York District Hospital, Wigginton Road, York YO3 7HE. Tel. 0904 31313.

Useful addresses

Active Birth Centre, International Centre for Active Birth, 55 Dartmouth Park Road, London, NW5 1SL. Tel. 01 267 3006.

Association for Improvements in the Maternity Services (AIMS), 21 Iver Lane, Iver, Buckinghamshire, SL0 9LH. Tel. 0753 652781.

Association of Radical Midwives (ARM), The Coppice, Greetby Hill, Ormskirk, Lancashire, L39 2DT. Tel. 0695 72776.

Birth Rights, c/o 2 Forth Street, Edinburgh, EH1 3LD. Tel. 031 667 5701 (N. Edinburgh); 031 557 0960 (S. Edinburgh).

Birthworks, Adam House, Adams Hill, Clent, West Midlands, DY9 9PS. Tel. 0562 883297.

British Holistic Medical Association, 179 Gloucester Place, London, NW1 6DX. Tel. 01 262 5299.

Health Education Authority (HEA), Third Floor, Hamilton House, Mableton Place, London, WC1A 9TX. Tel. 01 631 0930.

Health Rights, 344 South Lambeth Road, London, SW8 1UQ. Tel. 01 720 8911/2.

Home Birth Centre, 14 Marceuse Fields, Bosham, West Sussex, PO18 8NA. Tel. 0243 575066.

Independent Midwives Association (IMA), 65 Mount Nod Road, London, SW16 2LP. Tel. 01 677 9746.

Maternity Alliance, 15 Britannia Street, London, WC1X 9JP. Tel 01 837 1265.

Maternity Link, Old Co-op, 42 Chelsea Road, Easton, Bristol, BS5 6AF. Tel. 0272 541487.

Midwives Information and Resource Service
(MIDIRS)   Institute of Child Health, Royal Sick Children's
Hospital St. Michael's Hill, Bristol, BS2 8BJ. Tel. 0272 251791.

National Childbirth Trust (NCT),   Alexandra House, Oldham
Terrace, London, W3 6NH. Tel. 01 992 8637.

Parent Educators Group Support (PEGS),   c/o Royal College of
Midwives, (see below).

Rights of Women (ROW)   52–54 Featherstone Street, London,
EC1Y 8RT. Tel. 01 251 6577.

Royal College of Midwives (RCM)   15 Mansfield Road, London,
W1M 0BE. Tel. 01 580 6523.

Society to Support Home Confinements,   Lydgate, Lydgate
Lane, Wolsingham, DL13 3HA. Tel. 0388 528044.

Women's Health and Reproductive Rights Information Centre
(WHRRIC),   52–54 Featherstone Street, London, EC1. Tel. 01
251 6332.

References

Introduction

1. Richards, M. P. M. (1978). A place of safety? An examination of the risks of hospital delivery. In *Place of Birth*, Kitzinger, S. and Davis, J. A. (eds). Oxford University Press, Oxford.
2. Kitzinger, S. (1978). *Women as Mothers*, p. 105. W. Collins, Glasgow.
3. Donnison, J. (1979). The role of the midwife. *Association of Radical Midwives Newsletter*, Vol. 4 (June).
4. Calder, A. A. and Embrey, M. P. (1975). The management of labour. *Proceedings of the Royal College of Obstetricians and Gynaecologists Third Study Group*, Vol. 64.
5. Pincus, J. and Swenson, N. (1985). Boston Women's Health Collective. Introduction. In *Birthrights*, Inch, S., Pantheon, New York.
6. Raine, C. (1976). Look! Watch with father: a birth chronicled. *The Sunday Times*, 14 March 1976, p. 44.
7. Richards, M. P. M. (1977). Talk given to the Oxford Postnatal Support Group.
8. Senden, I. P. M., *et al.* (1988). Labour pain: a comparison of parturients in a Dutch and an American teaching hospital. *Obstetrics and Gynaecology*, Vol. 74 No. 4, pp. 541–4.

Chapter 1

1. Williams, A. and Reilly, W. (1988). Keep fit in pregnancy (short reports). *Nursing Times*, 20/26 July, p. 54.
2. Schwarcz, R. *et al.* (1974). Third progress report on the Latin

American Collaborative study on the effects of late rupture of the membranes on labour and the neonate. Submitted to the Director of the Pan-American Health Organization (PAHO) and the participating groups, Latin American Centre of Perinatology and Human Development, Montevideo, 1974. Reported in *Modern Perinatal Medicine*, Gluck, L. (ed.), p. 435. Year Book Medical Publishers, Chicago.

3. Mathie, J. G. and Dawson, B. H. (1959). Effect of castor oil, soap enema, and hot bath on the pregnant human uterus near term. *British Medical Journal*, 2 May, pp. 1162–5.

4. Schwarcz, R. (1974). As ref. 2, but p. 432.

5. Schwarcz, R., Diaz, A. G., Fescina, R., and Caldeyro-Barcia, R. (1979). Latin American Collaborative Study on Maternal Position in Labour. *Birth and the Family Journal*, Vol. 6, No. 1, pp. 7–15.

6. Odent, M. (1984). *Birth Reborn*. Pantheon, New York, pp. 12–13.

7. Fergusson, J. K. W. (1941). A study of the motility of the intact uterus at term. *Surgical Gynaecology and Obstetrics*, Vol. 73, pp. 359–66.

8. Greenspoon, J. S. and Paul, R. H. (1986). Paraplegia and quadriplegia: special considerations during pregnancy, labour and delivery. *American Journal of Obstetrics and Gynaecology*, Vol. 155, No. 4, pp. 738–41.

9. Naroll, F., Naroll, R., and Howard, F. H. (1961). Positions of women in childbirth. *American Journal of Obstetrics and Gynaecology*, Vol. 82, pp. 943–954.

10. Odent, M. (1987). The fetus ejection reflex. *Birth*, Vol. 14, No. 2, pp. 104–5.

11. Newton, N. (1987). The fetus ejection reflex revisited. *Birth*, Vol. 14, No. 2, pp. 106–8.

12. Dunn, P. M. (1966). Postnatal placental respiration. *Developmental Medicine and Child Neurology*, Vol. 8, No. 5, pp. 607–8.

13. Dunn, P. M. (1985). Management of childbirth in normal women: the third stage and fetal adaptation. In *Perinatal Medicine*, Clinch, J. and Matthews, T. (eds)., p. 50. Proceedings of the ninth European congress of perinatal medicine, Dublin, September 1984. MTP Press, Lancaster.

14. Ladipo, O. A. (1972). Management of the third stage of labour, with particular reference to reduction of feto-maternal transfusion. *British Medical Journal*, Vol. 1, pp. 721–3.

15. Botha, M. G. (1968). The management of the umbilical cord in Labour. *South African Journal of Obstetrics and Gynaecology*, Vol. 6 No. 2, pp. 30–3.

16. Walsh, S. Z. (1968). Maternal effects of early and late clamping of the umbilical cord. *Lancet*, Vol. i, pp. 966–7.

17. Mead, M. and Newton, N. (1967). Cultural patterning of perinatal behaviour. In *Childbearing: its Social and Psychological Aspects*. Richardson, S. A. and Guttmacher, A. F. (eds). Williams and Wilkins, Baltimore.

18. Ford, C. S. (1945). A comparative study of human reproduction. Yale University publications in anthropology, No. 32. Yale University Press, New Haven.

19. Widstrom, A. M. *et al.* (1987). Gastric suction in healthy newborn infants: effects on circulation and developing feeding behaviour. *Acta Paediatrica Scandinavica*, Vol. 76, pp. 566–72.

Chapter 2

1. Dick-Read, G. (1968). *Childbirth without Fear*, pp. 62–4. Pan Books, London.

2. Senden, I. M. P. *et al.* (1988). Labour pain, a comparison of parturients in a Dutch and American teaching hospital. *Obstetrics and Gynaecology*, Vol. 7, pp. 541–4.

3. McCammon, C. S. (1951). A study of 475 pregnancies in American-Indian women. *American Journal of Obstetrics and Gynaecology*, Vol. 61, pp. 1159–66.

4. Hommel, F. (1979). Can childbirth be painless? In *Emotion and Reproduction*, Carenza, L. and Zichella, L. (eds). Academic Press, London.

5. Davenport-Slack, B. and Boylan, C. H. (1974). Psychological correlates of childbirth pain. *Psychosomatic Medicine*, Vol. 36, pp. 215–23.

6. Melzack, R., Taenzer, P., Feldman, P. and Kinch, R. H. (1981). Labour is still painful after prepared childbirth training. *Canadian Medical Association Journal*, Vol. 125, pp. 357–63.

7. Balaskas, J. and Balaskas, A. (1979). *New Life*, London. pp. 100–1, Sedgwick and Jackson.

8. Shabanah, E. H., Toth, A. and Maughan, G. B. (1964). The role of the automatic nervous system in uterine contractility and bloodflow. *American Journal of Obstetrics and Gynaecology*, Vol. 89 No. 7, pp. 841–59.

9. Newton, N., Peeler, D. and Newton, M. (1968). Effect of

disturbance on labour: an experiment with 100 mice with dated pregnancies. *American Journal of Obstetrics and Gynaecology*, Vol. 101, pp. 1096–102.

10. Naaktegeboren, C. (1975). In *Immaculate deception*, Arms, S., pp. 130–2. Houghton Mifflin, Boston.

11. Janis, I. L. (1974). Vigilance and decision making in personal crises. In Coelho, G. V., Hamburg, D. A. and Adams, J. E. (eds). *Coping and Adaptation*. Basic Books, New York.

12. Crawford, M. I. (1968). Psychological and behavioural cues and disturbances in childbirth. *Bulletin of Sloane Hospital for Women*, Vol. 14, pp. 132–42.

13. Hott, J. R. (1980). Best laid plans. *Nursing Research*, Vol. 29, pp. 20–7.

14. Schwartz, R., Diaz, A. G., Fescina, R. and Caldeyro-Barcia, R. (1979). Latin American collaborative study on maternal position in labour, 1977. Reported in *Birth and the Family Journal*, Vol. 6 No. 1, pp. 7–16.

15. Mendez-Bauer, C. J. *et al.* (1976). Influences of maternal position on moulding and duration of labour. *Journal of Perinatal Medicine*, Vol. 3, p. 8–9.

16. Dunn, P. M. (1978). Posture in labour. *Lancet*, Vol. i, p. 496.

17. Flynn, A. M., Kelly, J., Hollins, G. and Lynch, P. F. (1978). Ambulation in labour. *British Medical Journal*, Vol. 2, pp. 591–3.

18. Gupta, J. and Liford, R. J. (1987). Birth positions. *Midwifery*, Vol. 3 No. 2, pp. 92–6.

19. Morgan, B. M., Bulpitt, C. J., Clifton, P. and Lewis, P. J. (1982). Analgesia and satisfaction in childbirth. The Queen Charlotte's 1000-mother survey. *Lancet*, Vol. 2, pp. 808–10.

20. Kitzinger, S. (1987). *Some Women's Experiences of Epidural Anaesthesia*. Available from: the National Childbirth Trust (see Useful Addresses).

21. Charles, A. G., Norr, K. L., Block, C. R., Meyering, S. and Meyers, E. (1978). Obstetric and psychological effects of psychoprophylactic preparation for childbirth. *American Journal of Obstetrics and Gynecology*, Vol. 131, pp. 44–52.

22. Zax, M., Sameroff, A. J. and Farnum, J. E. (1975). Childbirth education, maternal attitudes and delivery. *American Journal of Obstetrics and Gynecology*, Vol. 123 No. 2, pp. 185–90.

23. Brant, H. A. (1962). Childbirth with preparation and support in labour: an assessment. *New Zealand Medical Journal*, Vol. 61 No. 356, pp. 211–19.

24. Enkin, M. W., Smith, S. L., Derner, S. W. and Emmett, J. O.

(1972). An adequately controlled study of the effectiveness of PPM training. In *Psychosomatic Medicine in Obstetrics and Gynaecology*, Morris, N. (ed.). S. Kargar, Basel, pp. 62–67.

25. Huttel, F. A., Mitchell, I., Fischer, W. M. and Meyer, A. E. (1972). A quantitative evaluation of psycho-prophylaxis in childbirth. *Journal of Psychosomatic Research*, Vol. 16, pp. 81–93.
26. Timm, M. M. (1979). Prenatal education evaluation. *Nursing Research*, Vol. 28, pp. 338–42.
27. Ulrich, R. (1984). The view through a window may influence recovery from surgery. *Science*, Vol. 224, pp. 420–1.
28. O'Driscoll, K. (1975). An obstetricians's view of pain. *British Journal of Anaesthetics*, Vol. 47, pp. 1053–9.
29. Sosa, R., Kennell, J., Klaus, M., Robertson, S and Urrutia, J. (1980). The effect of a supportive companion on perinatal problems, length of labour, and mother-infant interaction. New England Journal of Medicine, Vol. 303, pp. 597–600.
30. Klein, M. *et. al.* (1983). A comparison of low-risk pregnant women booked for delivery in two systems of care. *British Journal of Obstetrics and Gynaecology*, Vol. 90, pp. 118–28.
31. Flint, C. and Poulengeris, P. (1987). *The 'Know your Midwife' Report*. A randomized controlled trial of continuity of care. Available from 49 Peckarmans Wood, Sydenham Hill, London, SE26 6RZ.

Chapter 3

1. *Pears Encyclopaedia* 1983–4, 92nd edn. Cook, C. and Barker, M. (eds), p. F29. Pelham Books Ltd, London.
2. Macfarlane, A. (1985). Reported in: Inch, S., Statistics and Policy making in the maternity services. *Journal of the Royal Society of Medicine*, Vol. 78, pp. 957–63.
3. Macfarlane, A. and Mugford, M. (1984). Birth Counts— statistics of pregnancy and childbirth, Vol. 2, p. 205. HMSO Publications, London.
4. Allen, E. L. (1966). *Guidebook to Western thought*. pp. 138–9. The English Universities Press. London.
5. Wagner, M. (1985). Filling the (w)holes in health. Paper presented at the British holistic Medical Association's second annual conference, 29–30 September 1984. (Available from the BHMA. See Useful Addresses.)
6. Savage, W. (1985). Reported in Inch, S., Attitudes of

obstetricians and midwives: a neglected area of study? *Journal of the Royal Society of Medicine*, Vol. 78, pp. 683–6.

7. Grant, A. and Mohide, P. (1982). Screening and diagnostic tests in antenatal care. In *Effectiveness and Satisfaction in Antenatal Care*, Enkin, M. and Chalmers, I. (eds), pp. 25 and 54. SIMP Heinemann Medical Books, London.

8. Hall, M. H., Chng, P. K. and MacGillivray, I. (1980). Is routine antenatal care worthwhile? *Lancet*, Vol. i, pp. 78–80.

9. Yudkin, P., Frumar, A. M., Anderson, A. M. B. and Turnbull, A. C. A retrospective study of Induction of Labour. *British Journal of Obstetrics and Gynaecology*, Vol. 86 No. 4, pp. 257–65.

10. Hoult, I. J., MacLennan, A. H. and Carrie, L. E. S. (1977). Lumbar epidural analgesia in labour: relation to fetal malposition and instrumental delivery. *British Medical Journal*, Vol. 1, pp. 14–16.

11. Banta, D. and Thacker, S. (1979). Electronic fetal monitoring: is it of benefit? *Birth and the Family Journal*, Vol. 6 No. 4, pp. 237–49.

12. Inch, S. (1982). *Birthrights*, p. 244. Hutchinson, London.

Chapter 4

1. Richards, M. P. M. (1981). Whose choice in childbirth?, pp. 7–13. Paper presented at the National Childbirth Trust Silver Jubilee, and subsequently published by the NCT, (see Useful Addresses).

2. Huntingford, P. (1981). Choice in childbirth, pp. 4–6. NCT Silver Jubilee, as ref. 1.

3. Campbell, R. and Macfarlane, A. (1987). *Where to be Born—the Debate and the Evidence*. Published by and obtainable from: National Perinatal Epidemiology Unit, Radcliffe Infirmary, Oxford OX2 6HE.

4. Tew, M. (1985). Place of birth and perinatal mortality. *Journal of the Royal College of General Practitioners* vol. 35, pp. 390–3.

5. Marsh, G. N. (1977). Obstetric audit in General Practice. *British Medical Journal*, vol. 2, pp. 1004–6.

6. Taylor, G. W. (1980). How safe is general practitioner obstetrics? *Lancet*, vol. ii, pp. 1287–9.

7. Black, N. (1982). Do general practitioner deliveries constitute a perinatal mortality risk? *British Medical Journal*, No. 284, pp. 488–90.

8. Rosenblatt, R. A. (1985). Is obstetrics safe in small hospitals? *Lancet*, Vol. ii. pp. 429–31.

9. Campbell, R., Davies, I. M., Macfarlane, A. and Beral, V.

(1984). Home births in England and Wales, 1979; perinatal mortality according to intended place of delivery. *British Medical Journal*, Vol. 289, pp. 721–4.

10. Klein, M. and Zander, L. The role of the family practitioner. In *Effective Care in Pregnancy and Childbirth*. Enkin, M., Keirse, M. and Chalmers, I. (eds). Oxford University Press, Oxford (in press).

11. Rosen, M., Payne, J. (1985). Pain-free childbirth—how safe is it? *The Times*, 1 February 1985.

12. Riley, E. M. D. (1977). What do women want? The question of choice in the conduct of labour. In: *Benefits and Hazards of the New Obstetrics*, Chard, T. and Richards, M. P. M. (eds), pp. 62–71. SIMP Heinemann Medical Books, London.

13. Goodlin, R. C. (1980). Low-risk obstetric care for low-risk mothers. *Lancet*, Vol. ii, pp. 1017–19.

14. Mehl, L. (1976). Home vs hospital delivery; comparison of matched populations. In *Place of Birth*, Kitzinger, S. and Davis, J. A. (eds), pp. 109–13. Oxford University Press, Oxford.

15. Klein, M., Lloyd, I., Redman, C., Bull, M. and Turnbull, A. C. (1983). A comparison of low-risk pregnant women booked for delivery in two systems of care: shared care (consultant) and integrated general practice unit. *British Journal of Obstetrics and Gynaecology*, Vol. 90, pp. 118–28.

16. Flint, C. and Poulengeris, P. (1987). *The Know Your Midwife Report*. Available from 49 Peckarmans Wood, Sydenham Hill, London SE26 6RZ.

17. Hickey, J. and Metcalfe, J. (1987). As reported in Inch, S., Care in labour—a need for re-assessment? *Journal of the Royal Society of Medicine*, Vol. 80, pp. 388–91.

18. Riley, E. M. D. (1977). As reported in Inch, S., Care in labour.

19. Kitzinger, S. (1984). *Some Mothers' Experiences of Induced Labour*. (Also Kitzinger and Walters: *Some Women's Experiences of Episiotomy*) Both available from The National Childbirth Trust (see Useful Addresses).

20. Kitzinger, S. (1987). *Some Women's Experiences of Epidurals*. Available from The National Childbirth Trust (see Useful Addresses).

21. Richards, M. P. M. (1981). See ref. 1.

22. Morgan, E. (1972). *The Descent of Woman*, p. 229. Corgi Books, London.

Chapter 5

1. Flint, C. (1986), *Sensitive Midwifery*, pp. 31–32. Heinemann Medical Books, London.
2. Shapiro, R. (1988). Domino Babies. *Good Housekeeping*, December 1988.
3. Janis, I. L. (1974). Vigilance and decision-making in personal crises. In *Coping and Adaptation*, Coelho, G. V., Hamburg, D. A. and Adams, J. E. (eds). Basic Books, New York.
4. Lumley, J. and Astbury, J. (1980). *Birth Rites, Birth Rights — Childbirth Alternatives for Australian Parents*, p.36. Sphere Books, Australia.
5. Odent, M. Personal communication. See also Odent, M., (1984) *Birth Reborn*, p. 24. Pantheon Books, New York.
6. Shachter, M. (1982). Modern approaches to the control of pain. *Geriatric Medicine*, January 1982, pp. 47–52.
7. Lumley, J. and Astbury, J. As ref. 4, but p. 53.
8. Inch, S. (1988). Birth plans and protocols. *Journal of the Royal Society of Medicine*, Vol. 81, pp. 120–2.
9. Dawley, K., Mesuse, M. and Keyes, M. (1982). *Childbirth Choices* and *Where to Go: Having a Baby in Philadelphia*. Both published by CHOICE, 1501 Cherry Street, Philadelphia, PA 19102, USA.
10. Kitzinger S. (1983). *The New Good Birth Guide*. Penguin Books, Harmondsworth.
11. Milner, I. (1986). Choosing a natural or active birth. *Nursing*, Vol. 3 No. 2, pp. 39–45.
12. Odent M. (1984). As ref. 5, but pp. 15–16.
13. Klein, M. (1983). Contracting for trust in family practice obstetrics. *Canadian Family Physician*, Vol. 29, pp. 2225–7.

Appendix 1

1. Moore, W. O. M. (1978). In *Place of Birth*, Kitzinger S. and David, J. (eds), p. 4. Oxford University Press, Oxford. Unless otherwise referenced, all the 'indicators of risk' are taken from this book.
2. *Williams Obstetrics*, 16th edn (1981), p. 759. Pritchard J. A. MacDonald P. C. Appleton-Century—Crofts, New York.
3. Odell, L. D. and Mengert, W. F. (1945). The overweight obstetric patient. *Journal of the American Medical Association*, Vol. 128 no. 2, pp. 87–9.
4. Maeder, E. C., Barno, A. and Mecklenburg, F. (1975). Obesity:

a maternal high-risk factor. *Obstetrics and Gynecology*, Vol. 45 no. 6, pp. 669–71.

5. Peckham, C. H. and Christianson, R. A. (1971). The relationship between prepregnancy weight and certain obstetric factors. *American Journal of Obstetrics and Gynecology*, Vol. 111, No. 1, pp. 1–7.

6. Edwards, L. E., Dickes, W. F., Alton, I. R. and Hakanson, E. Y. (1978). Pregnancy in the massively obese: course, outcome and obesity prognosis of the infant. *American Journal of Obstetrics and Gynecology*, Vol 131. No. 5, pp. 479–83.

7. Harrison, G. G., Udall, J. N. and Morrow, G. (1980). Maternal obesity, weight gain in pregnancy and infant birth weight. *American Journal of Obstetrics and Gynecology*, Vol. 136 No. 3, pp. 411–2.

8. Roopnarinesingh, S. S. and Pathak, U. N. (1970). Obesity in the Jamaican parturient. *Journal of Obstetrics and Gynecology*, Vol. 77, pp. 895–9.

9. Tracy, T. A. and Miller, G. L. (1969). Obstetric problems of the massively obese. *Obstetrics and Gynecology*, Vol. 33 No. 2, pp. 204–8.

10. Molloy, B. G., Sheil, O. and Duignan, N. M. (1987). Delivery after caesarean section: review of 2176 consecutive cases. *British Medical Journal* No. 294, p. 1645.

11. Hall, M., Halliwell, R. and Carr-Hill, R. (1985). Concomitant and repeated happenings of the third stage of labour. *British Journal of Obstetrics and Gynaecology*, Vol. 92, pp. 732–8.

12. Inch, S. (1985). Management of the third stage of labour—another cascade of intervention? *Midwifery*, Vol. 1. pp. 114–22.

13. Inch, S. (1988). Physiology of the third stage of labour. *Midwives Chronicle*. February 1988, pp. 42–3.

14. Hall, M., Chng, P. K. and MacGillivray, I. (1980). Is routine antenatal care worthwhile? *Lancet*, Vol. ii, pp. 78–80.

15. Niswander, K. R. and Gordon, M. (1972). *The Women and Their Pregnancies*, p. 126. Collaborative study of the National Institute of Neurological Diseases and Stroke. W. B. Saunders, Philadelphia.

Also by Sally Inch from Green Print

Birthrights

'The strength and originality of this book lie in the fact that Sally Inch brings together past and present research as no one else has yet done—and makes it accessible to us all. She has a knack for presenting the kind of information offered in medical journals and texts simply and clearly, combining it with commonsense observations about the actions and attitudes that enable women to feel most at ease during childbirth. Her tone is objective throughout, but her underlying passion for the truth and her respect for women are evident in her systematic presentation of medical and sociological findings and in her assurance that it is possible—indeed necessary—to make hard facts about childbirth in hospitals available to everyone concerned.

'By giving us the facts, *Birthrights* enables us to combat the charge that our opposition to many routine procedures is mere superstition, paranoia or emotionalism. It helps us to define the limits of childbirth technology so that it can work for us without harming us. Above all, it confirms our conviction that it is we ourselves who must do this work of warning and explaining, for neither those who have the power to introduce and use these tools, nor those who stand to profit most from their use, will do it for us.'

Quotation from Jane Pincus and Norma Swenson, in the foreword to the US edition of this book.

Re-issued with minor corrections, 1989
ISBN 1 85425 032 9   £7.99 paperback